Blood Banking and Regulation: Procedures, Problems, and Alternatives

Forum on Blood Safety and Blood Availability

Division of Health Sciences Policy

INSTITUTE OF MEDICINE

Edward A. Dauer, *Editor*

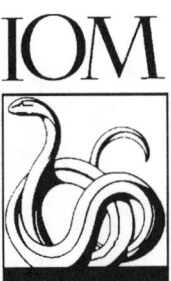

NATIONAL ACADEMY PRESS
Washington, D.C. 1996

National Academy Press • 2101 Constitution Avenue, NW • Washington, DC 20418

NOTICE: The project that oversees this report was approved by the Governing Board of the National Research Council, whose members are drawn from the councils of the National Academy of Science, the National Academy of Engineering, and the Institute of Medicine. The members of the forum responsible for this report were chosen for their special competencies and with regard for appropriate balance.

This report has been reviewed by a group other than the authors according to the procedures approved by a Report Review Committee consisting of members of the National Academy of Sciences, the National Academy of Engineering, and the Institute of Medicine.

The Institute of Medicine was chartered in 1970 by the National Academy of Sciences to enlist distinguished memers of the appropriate professions in the examination of policy matters pertaining to the health of the public. In this, the Institute acts under both the Academy's 1863 congressional charter responsibility to be an adviser to the federal government and its own initiative in identifying issues of medical care, research, and education. Dr. Kenneth I. Shine is president of the Institute of Medicine.

Support for this project was provided by the Food and Drug Administration (Contract No. 223-93-1025), Abbott Laboratories, Baxter Health Care Corporation, Ortho Diagnostic Systems, the American Association of Blood Banks, the American Red Cross, the American Blood Resources Association, and the Council of Community Blood Centers. This support does not consitute an endorsement of the views expressed in the report.

Library of Congress Catalog Card No. 96-69310
International Standard Book Number 0-309-05546-6

Additional copies of this report are available from: National Academy Press, Lock Box 285, 2101 Constitution Avenue, N.W., Washington, D.C. 20055.

Call (800) 624-6242 or (202) 334-3313 (in the Washington metropolitan area), or visit the NAP on-line bookstore at **http://www.nap.edu/nap/bookstore/**.

Call (202) 334-2352 for more information on the other activities of the Institute of Medicine, or visit the IOM home page at **http://www.nas.edu/iom/**.

Copyright 1996 by the National Academy of Sciences. All rights reserved.
Printed in the United States of America

The serpent has been a symbol of long life, healing, and knowledge among almost all cultures and religions since the beginning of recorded history. The image adopted as a logotype by the Institute of Medicine is based on a relief carving from ancient Greece, now held by the Staatlichemuseen in Berlin.

Cover design by Francesca Moghari.

FORUM ON BLOOD SAFETY AND BLOOD AVAILABILITY

HENRIK H. BENDIXEN, *Chair*, Professor Emeritus, Department of Anesthesiology, Columbia University, New York, New York.

THOMAS F. ZUCK, *Vice Chair*, Professor of Transfusion Medicine, University of Cincinnati, Director, Hoxworth Blood Center, Cincinnati, Ohio

JOHN W. ADAMSON, President, New York Blood Center, New York, New York

ARTHUR L. CAPLAN, Director, Center for Bioethics, University of Pennsylvania, Philadelphia, Pennsylvania

WILLIAM COENEN,[*] Administrator, Community Blood Center of Greater Kansas City, Kansas City, Missouri

PINYA COHEN, Vice President of Quality Assurance and Regulatory Affairs, NABI, Boca Raton, Florida

EDWARD A. DAUER, Dean Emeritus, College of Law, University of Denver, Denver, Colorado

M. ELAINE EYSTER, Distinguished Professor of Medicine, Division of Hematology, The Milton Hershey Medical Center, Hershey, Pennsylvania

JOSEPH C. FRATANTONI, Director, Division of Hematology, Office of Blood Research and Review, Food and Drug Administration, Rockville, Maryland

HARVEY G. KLEIN, Chief, Department of Transfusion Medicine, Warren Grant Magnuson Clinical Center, National Institutes of Health, Bethesda, Maryland

EVE M. LACKRITZ, Medical Epidemiologist, HIV Seroepidemiology Branch, Division of HIV/AIDS, National Center for Infectious Diseases, Centers for Disease Control and Prevention, Atlanta, Georgia

PAUL R. McCURDY, Director, Blood Resources Program, National Heart, Lung, and Blood Institute, Bethesda, Maryland

PAUL S. RUSSELL, John Homans Professor of Surgery, Massachusetts General Hospital, Boston, Massachusetts

CAPT BRUCE D. RUTHERFORD, MSC, USN, Director, Armed Services Blood Program, Falls Church, Virginia

WILLIAM C. SHERWOOD, Director, Transfusion Services, American Red Cross Blood Services, Philadelphia, Pennsylvania

LINDA STEHLING, Director of Medical Affairs, Blood Systems, Inc., Scottsdale, Arizona

---

[*] Served from January 1995 until December 1995.

EUGENE TIMM,** Member, Board of Directors, American Blood Resources Association, Rochester Hill, Michigan

ROBERT M. WINSLOW, Adjunct Professor of Medicine, University of California-San Diego, and Hematology-Oncology Section, Veterans Affairs Medical Center, San Diego, California

Project Staff

VALERIE P. SETLOW, Director, Health Sciences Policy Division
FREDERICK J. MANNING, Project Director
KIMBERLY KASBERG MARAVIGLIA, Research Associate
MARY JANE BALL, Sr. Project Assistant
NANCY DIENER, Financial Associate (until March 1996)
JAMAINE TINKER, Financial Associate (after March 1996)

** Served from January 1994 until December 1994.

PRESENTERS

MICHAEL BEATRICE, Deputy Director, Center for Biologics Evaluation and Research, Food and Drug Administration, Bethesda, Maryland

JAY EPSTEIN, Director, Office of Blood Research and Review, Center for Biologics Evaluation and Research, Food and Drug Administration, Bethesda, Maryland

ANNE MARIE FINLEY, Professional Staff, House Government Reform and Oversight Committee, Subcommittee on Human Resources and Intergovernment Relations, Washington, DC

PHILIP HARTER, Attorney at Law, Washington, DC

MARY K. PENDERGAST, Deputy Commissioner and Senior Advisor to the Commissioner, Food and Drug Administration, Rockville, Maryland

LYLE PETERSEN, Chief, HIV Seroepidemiology Branch, Centers for Disease Control and Prevention, Atlanta, Georgia

DAVID PRITZKER, Senior Attorney, Regulatory Information Service Center, General Services Administration, Washington, DC

MERLYN SAYERS, Director of Transfusion Services, Puget Sound Blood Center, Seattle Washington

SIDNEY SHAPIRO, Rounds Professor of Law, University of Kansas School of Law, Lawrence, Kansas

JAMES C. SIMMONS, Director, Office of Compliance, Center for Biologics Evaluation and Research, Food and Drug Administration, Bethesda, Maryland

TOBY SIMON, President, Blood Systems Foundation, Scottsdale, Arizona

RICHARD SWANSON, Director, Division of Emergency and Investigative Operations, Office of Regional Operations, Food and Drug Administration, Rockville, Maryland

KATHRYN C. ZOON, Director, Center for Biologics Evaluation and Research, Food and Drug Administration, Bethesda, Maryland

Foreword

This is the first of three monographs by the Forum on Blood Safety and Blood Availability. Each monograph provides a review and summary of selected topical presentations at four separate workshops sponsored by the Forum from January 1994 through September 1995. The talks summarized in this document were originally given at workshops on Alterative Regulatory Models (January, 1995); CBER Compliance Activity, Theory and Practice (September, 1995); and Managing Threats to the Blood Supply (September, 1995). The views expressed in this document, unless otherwise noted, are those of the individual presenters and do not reflect the views of the individual's employing agency or the Institute of Medicine. This document is neither a summary of any one workshop nor a comprehensive summary of all of the Forum's workshops. Rather, it is a compilation of talks that were specifically selected to provide a clear and comprehensive perspective of the current decision making and regulatory processes in the blood arena, as well as some alternative regulatory models that have been applied in other regulatory venues (i.e., air traffic control and environmental protection). To promote full participation by Forum members, presenters, and invited guests, the Forum does not draw conclusions or make recommendations.

The Forum on Blood Safety and Blood Availability was convened by the Institute of Medicine to provide an environment for the exchange of information about blood safety and blood availability, to identify high-priority issues in these areas, and to promote problem solving activities such as workshops. During its two years of existence, the Forum identified opportunities and problems that are ongoing or expected to arise within the next five years, and has developed approaches to exploiting opportunities or solving problems.

During the Forum's final meeting, in September 1995, members of the Forum reviewed its work and addressed the question of how the dialogue that it had fostered might best be continued or improved. One of the questions the group considered was what the criteria should be for any such future venture. Not everyone agreed with everything mentioned, and no votes were taken; consistent with its charter, the Forum reached no specific conclusions or recommendations. The group did, however, request that the collected list of criteria be recorded as a possible starting point for any subsequent initiative. The suggestions on that list included the following "Criteria for a Process of Dialogue:"

1. A consensus oriented procedure capable of reaching closure on the issues being discussed.
2. Participation of diverse constituencies, such as designated representatives of the public.
3. Continuity of people and process, so that issues may be addressed as they arise without the need to fashion a structure and process ad hoc.
4. Conditions supporting openness and candor.
5. Opportunities for discussion in a variety of venues, both public and—where permitted by law—private.
6. Prestigious and neutral, a forum that lends dignity and credibility to the discussions.
7. Expert facilitation, though not necessarily subject-matter expertise, by those who run or manage the process.
8. Less time devoted to education about the issues, allowing more direct engagement with decision-making.
9. Available and ready to be utilized whenever an appropriate issue is identified.
10. Fashioned to be persuasive to Congress and others.

Preface

The Forum on Blood Safety and Blood Availability was convened by the Institute of Medicine in the spring of 1994 with the objective of providing a forum within which representatives of blood banking and transfusion medicine, representatives of the Food and Drug Administration (FDA) and other government agencies, and interested members of the public could meet to discuss informally and freely questions of common interest. That common interest was defined to be the safety and availability of the nation's supply of blood and blood components.

It became apparent early in the course of the Forum's meetings that the topic of *regulation* should have a place on the agenda. Regulation may be taken formally to mean the method by which government authority shapes the activities of firms and organizations in the private sector, in accordance with policy directives established by the legislative and executive branches of the federal government. Less formally, but of equal importance in a field like blood banking, which operates in the public interest and where the expertise required for good decision-making lies as much outside government as within it, regulatory methods are among the vehicles by which that expertise is shared and applied to the issues that both the public and private sectors face. Particularly in recent years, questions had been raised about the ways in which both the formal and less formal functions of regulation had been working.

At the same time, developments in alternative forms of regulation in general had progressed quite markedly. "Negotiated Rule-making," for example, was formally sanctioned and encouraged by a federal statute enacted in 1990. During the early 1990s, the Administrative Conference of the United States, then a federal agency service office, supported several experiments in regulatory alternatives, many of them notably successful. Field experience with and a mature literature about the new techniques were being developed, and individuals in the upper levels of the Executive Branch had itself taken note of these alternative models.

These two streams converged: the sense among some in blood banking, inside government and out, that the regulatory process could profitably undergo some deliberate reconsideration, and the emergence of demonstrated alternative techniques for government regulation. The Forum therefore devoted a significant portion of its working time to the exploration of these questions: How well does the present regulatory system work? Are there alternatives that hold promise for enhancing its functions?

The principal discussions of regulation and alternative regulation occurred during the Forum session of January 1995. The ideas advanced at that time generated additional questions and suggestions, resulting in a further discussion among Forum members at their meeting in June 1995. The meeting in September 1995 included several segments of closely related material, specifically the enforcement side of regulation and the role and direction of congressional oversight of blood safety and availability. This report includes selections from each of those three meetings, but they are rearranged to create a more continuous sequence.

The usual way of proceeding at the Forum meetings was through panel discussions. One or more speakers would offer an initial set of prepared remarks. This would be followed by a period of open discussion among the speakers and the Forum members and guests. The principal selections included in this report are edited versions of the speakers' presentations. They have been edited to change the patterns of an oral presentation into the more readable patterns of a written text, and in a few instances they have been edited for length. No effort has been made to integrate or summarize the individual presentations. In each case the views expressed are those of the individual speaker and not those of the Forum or the Institute of Medicine.

Although the discussion sessions were in many senses the greatest success of the Forum meetings, they required more extensive editing to create a text that was readable rather than one that jumped abruptly from one subject to the next. The give and take of an open discussion does not always translate well when reported verbatim. In some places in this report a question put to a speaker, and its answer, may be reported in full; in other cases, the editor has taken the liberty of combining related aspects of the discussion into a composite narrative. Although some of the liveliness may thus be subdued, it is hoped that the accessibility of the subject to the reader will have been improved.

Edward A. Dauer

Contents

I Overview of Regulatory and Policy-Making Procedures in Blood Banking 1
FDA Policy and Regulation, *Michael Beatrice*, 3
CDC Recommendations, *Lyle Petersen*, 9
Blood Banking's Policy Groups and Procedures, *Toby Simon*, 13
Opportunities and Venues for Dialogue, *Merlyn Sayers*, 19
Discussion, 25

II Regulatory Enforcement and Compliance 27
CBER Compliance Activity, *James Simmons*, 29
FDA Practice in the Field, *Richard Swanson*, 33
Challenges and Questions About Compliance, *William Sherwood*, 35
Discussion, 41

III Innovations and Alternatives in Regulation 47
Regulatory Alternatives, *Sidney Shapiro*, 49
Specific Techniques, *David Pritzker*, 55
Negotiated Rule-Making, *Philip Harter*, 61
Panel Discussion on Applications of Negotiated Rule-Making to Issues in Blood Banking,
    Kathryn C. Zoon, 73
    Jay Epstein, 76
    Toby Simon, 81
General Discussion of Issues for Negotiated Rule-Making, 87

IV Congressional Oversight and Regulatory Initiatives 91
Congressional Oversight of Blood Safety Issues, *Anne Marie Finley*, 93
DHHS Task Force on HIV and the Blood Supply, *Mary Pendergast*, 99

V Postscript **103**
   Investing in Regulatory Quality, *Edward A. Dauer*, 105

Appendixes **107**
A Negotiated Rule-Making Procedure, 109
B Workshop Participants, 121
C Acronyms, 125

I

Overview of Regulatory and Policy-Making Procedures in Blood Banking

FDA Policy and Regulation

Michael Beatrice

The Food and Drug Administration (FDA) is presently re-examining its regulatory mechanisms in an effort to do more with less. At the same time, matters relating to blood products and blood services are under intense scrutiny by the public. The discussion of regulatory alternatives is therefore quite timely.

THE REGULATORY MANDATE

The Center for Biologics Evaluation and Research (CBER) is that part of FDA responsible for regulating blood, plasma, and other biological products such as banked human tissue, somatic cells, stem cells, vaccines, allergenic products, and various biological therapeutics. Recently, the Blood and Blood Components Review Program was reorganized by combining the Division of Blood Product and Establishment Applications and Review Policy with the Division of Blood Collection and Processing. This change, accomplished in February 1994, was intended to streamline the review process.

CBER operates on the assumption that the public—including the scientific and the professional public—expects more than a passive regulatory bureaucracy. This philosophy and the involvement that CBER has with various components of the blood services complex have made the center a more effective partner in bringing about constructive change and regulation. Regulation should be a thoughtful blend of medical needs, statutory authority, and public expectation. When logic and scientific thinking indicate that there is a need for change, it is the responsibility of the center to find a mechanism to bring about that change.

Protection of the public health requires active facilitation, as well as the more traditional restrictive components of regulation. The availability of blood and new and improved blood products, for example, is fully as important as the elimination of poor practices in processing and manufacture. If FDA is to work effectively, it must understand the need for productive interactions with many groups in translating basic scientific data into medical and manufacturing practice.

REGULATORY MECHANISMS

CBER has a number of tools available to it to pursue its mission. One of them is the *technical workshop*, a natural outgrowth of scientist-to-scientist communication that can result in the issuance of guidelines by FDA for the industry. Recent technical workshops have been on topics of gene amplification technology, to close the window of human immunodeficiency virus infectivity; hemoglobin substitutes; computer validation of blood quality assurance; evaluation of the interim regulations for banked human tissue; and viral inactivation methods to reduce infectivity in plasma products. Additional workshops being planned cover blood licensing and methods of leukocyte reduction in blood components. In these workshops FDA expects to receive input from the industry on regulatory issues, as well as to educate the industry about its standards and guidelines.

Another mechanism is the *advisory committee*, which often is of use in assisting the agency in reaching a regulatory decision. As of January 1995, there were four such advisory committees, each of which comprised physicians, scientists, biostatisticians, and others. The committees provide scientific and medical opinions, and elicit for the agency's consideration public comment on the safety, effectiveness, and appropriate use of the products under CBER's jurisdiction.

Several methods of providing regulations and guidance are available. They range from proposed formal *regulations*, which have their origins with the publication of a notice and invitation to comment in the *Federal Register*, to the issuance of *guidelines* and *"points to consider,"* which are documents for the more rapid dissemination of current information. Regulations are binding on both FDA and the industry. Guidelines may be binding if they are recognized as industry standards. "Points to consider" are always regarded as draft documents, subject to revision as additional comments are received.

A related mechanism that is also used to indicate agency practice and expectations the is the use of *recommendations*, which are usually in the form of memoranda to manufacturers. Although these memoranda are not regulations, they are based on regulations and may be issued when necessary as interpretive or explanatory documents to achieve rapid communication with the industry.

LEGAL AUTHORITIES

The authority under which blood and plasma are regulated has changed over the years. Today's laws regulating drugs and biological products (biologics) are administered in a coordinated manner, even though they were drafted, passed, and implemented separately. Among the earliest were the Biologics Control Act of 1902, also called the Virus, Serum and Toxins Act, and the Pure Food and Drugs Act of 1906, which established purity standards for food and drugs.

Because early vaccines and antitoxins were then administered by direct injection, as compared with drugs, which were largely ingested, legislation related to biologics occurred earlier and was stricter than that for drugs from the outset. The production of biologics requires a licensing process, as it did in 1902 and so does today. With licensing came inspections. In 1902 licensed establishments were inspected by scientists and medical officers from the National Hygienic Laboratory, the forerunner of the present National Institutes of Health (NIH).

Today, biologics are also defined as drugs. Therefore, when the biological authorities joined FDA in 1972, all of the provisions of the federal Food, Drug and Cosmetic Act (FD&C Act) became operative. Having the authority to administer both the FD&C Act and the Public Health Service Act (PHS Act) now gives FDA great flexibility and scope.

The laws dealing with food and drugs originally dealt only with purity, not with safety and efficacy. The drugs act was strengthened in 1938 with the birth of the federal FD&C Act, which included safety along with purity.

The ensuing years saw consolidations and reorganizations. In 1944 the Virus, Serum and Toxin Act was consolidated with other laws into the PHS Act; and in 1948 biologics regulation was focused in the new National Microbiological Institute. By that time the first blood bank, the Philadelphia Blood Bank, had been licensed, and biologics authorities embarked on the licensing of whole blood and blood derivatives. In 1955 the responsibility for biologics regulation was transferred from the National Microbiologics Institute (now the National Institute of Allergy and Infectious Diseases) to an independent division of the called the Division of Biologic Standards.

REGULATION AND ENFORCEMENT AT FDA

The Division of Biologic Standards, the DBS as it was known, was transferred to FDA in 1972 and became the Bureau of Biologics. It has remained in FDA ever since, with occasional variations in its size, structure, and affiliations. Today it is an organization with more than 800 scientists, medical officers, and support personnel. Its three offices for product review have full authority to review products, from the investigational stage through marketing.

The Office of Blood Research and Review currently has a staff of 105 organized into three divisions: the Division of Transfusion Transmitted Diseases, the Division of Hematology, and the Division of Blood Applications.

In an earlier day, when the number of licensed blood banks was less than 150 and antibody identification panels were considered high technology, the regulatory climate could best be described as relaxed. Relationships with manufacturers, including blood bank personnel, were professional but collegial. As one commentator observed, "It is not surprising that . . . [being] led by medical personnel whose primary mission was public health rather than law enforcement, a laboratory of blood and blood products of the Division of Biologic Standards carried out the administration of biologic law in the manner of communication among physicians."

This environment changed dramatically with the first prosecution of an individual in a commercial blood bank in 1962. The responsible head of the blood bank was found guilty of falsification of records, mislabeling, and adulteration and was permanently barred from practicing blood banking in any licensed facility. The Justice Department at the time elected to prosecute the case under both the drug and the biologics statutes, since prior to that time the courts had held that blood was not a biological product because it was not enumerated specifically in the PHS Act. In 1973 the PHS Act was amended to include blood explicitly.

The more frequent administrative actions against a license include revocation or suspension. A license may be revoked at the request of the licensee for various reasons such as the discontinuation of the manufacture of the product. In instances in which manufacturers waive the opportunity for a hearing and request revocation, the revocation is without prejudice.

Licenses may also be revoked for cause, such as a failure to allow FDA access to facilities, failure to report in advance significant changes to products or facilities, failure to conform to applicable standards in the license, changes in the manufacturing methods that require a new showing, or producing a licensed product that is not safe and effective for all of its intended uses.

The agency may initiate a revocation in either of two ways. It may issue a notice of intent to revoke, which allows a firm the opportunity to demonstrate or achieve compliance within a reasonable period of time. Or the agency may inform the firm of its intention to move directly to revocation, without allowing time for the firm to demonstrate or achieve compliance. The latter course is usually indicated when the violations are considered willful, such as intentional record falsification.

Notices of intent to revoke have been issued for documented, repeated significant variations from good manufacturing practices after prior warnings have already been given. FDA may also suspend a license if the Commissioner has reason to believe that one or more grounds for license revocation exists *and* if a danger to health exists. In such a case the license is immediately suspended, preventing the products from being shipped interstate.

Another remedy available to the agency is the voluntary recall, which is used for products in violation of the laws administered by FDA. Recalls may be initiated by manufacturers or distributors or at the request of FDA. FDA-requested recalls are usually reserved for urgent situations, for example, when a firm refuses to undertake a recall requested by FDA, when FDA has reason to believe that a voluntary recall would not be effective, or when violations are continuing and it is necessary to seize the product.

A more radical remedy is a seizure, a civil action taken against a product designed to remove it from the market quickly. Products are not seized without prior warning unless there is documented harm to the consumer from their continued use.

Similarly, an injunction may be requested from a court to stop or prevent a violation of the law and to correct the conditions that caused the violation to occur again. Appropriate prior notice is required, and the injunction is generally sought only after the agency comes to believe that no other steps will stop the continuing violation.

Other types of regulatory actions can follow from inspections of manufacturing facilities. Again, biologics facilities are licensed under authority of the PHS Act, and since they are also drugs, the facilities that manufacture them are also inspected under the authority of the FD&C Act.

A preapproval or prelicense inspection is conducted prior to the approval of a facility. Once approved, each facility is inspected on a regular basis thereafter. Since 1988, the inspections have been annual. The results of the inspection, including observations, deficiencies, and violations, are given to the individual responsible for the facility—usually the "responsible head." The report lists the observations that are significant enough to require a response or a corrective action. If the observations are of sufficient magnitude or if they continue after substantial notice has been given, the agency may issue a warning letter specifying the violations and threatening additional legal action if the problems are not addressed within a short time, usually 30 days.

Pre-approval inspections are conducted by Center personnel experienced in the review of applications for blood processing facilities. The postapproval annual inspections are done by personnel in the field.

ENSURING BLOOD SAFETY AND AVAILABILITY IN THE FUTURE

The future of blood safety and availability lies at least partly in technical innovation. Advances in testing, such as gene amplification, may yield better sensitivity. Hemoglobin- and non-hemoglobin-based blood substitutes may also be developed, as may recombinant and other molecular techniques for producing substitutes for products now derived from blood. Better methods of evaluating donor safety and recruitment are also being investigated, and as important as scientific advances are, there may be even more potential in donor recruitment and systems efficiency.

From a regulatory perspective, strategies must be developed by FDA and industry to provide quality assurance, to prevent errors and accidents, and to ensure conformance with legal requirements without losing the identity of blood banks as both a needed medical service and as manufacturers of biological products. This will require the development of more meaningful partnerships between the federal government and the private sector and between the public and members of the health professions.

CDC Recommendations

Lyle Petersen

CDC'S MISSION

The mission of the Centers for Disease Control and Prevention (CDC) is to be the national leader in disease prevention and control in the United States. It serves this mission partly through public health-related research, facilitated by a unique integration among epidemiology, statistics, and laboratory science. That research provides the basis for CDC's voluntary guidelines and recommendations. CDC also provides consultation and assistance to federal agencies, state and local health departments, other nations, and international agencies. This consultation and assistance function has been notable in the blood arena, where CDC has provided data and expert opinion to the Food and Drug Administration (FDA).

EFFECTIVENESS OF CDC

The influence that CDC has in national health policy can be attributed to several factors. First, CDC is not a regulatory agency and has no regulatory authority, even though it does have a public health mandate. Thus, the only way that CDC can exert influence is to build consensus. Accordingly, the emphasis is on data-based decision-making and an intense effort at consensus building as the basis for its recommendations. Second, CDC enjoys a strongly positive public perception. Third, it has developed the ability to disseminate data and recommendations rapidly through scientific publications and, more importantly, through the *Morbidity and Mortality Weekly Report (MMWR)*.

RESEARCH ON HIV

Although many of CDC research efforts concentrate on the human immunodeficiency virus (HIV), they are applicable to other transfusion-transmissible diseases as well. In one such interview-based study funded by CDC, HIV-seropositive donors at 20 blood centers are interviewed for HIV risk factors, their motivations for donation, and other behavioral characteristics. CDC has also funded a national database with information from 19 American Red Cross blood centers, including all infectious disease marker, demographic, and donation history data. These investigations have proven vital for studying the risk of HIV transmission by transfusion. Another study of seroconverting blood donors has helped to define the "window period of infectivity. These activities occur in conjunction with ongoing investigations of disease outbreaks, including individual transfusion-associated instances of hepatitis as well as HIV.

Internationally, through a cooperative agreement with the U.S. Agency for International Development, CDC investigates the degree and quality of blood screening in other countries and assesses the feasibility of recruiting low-risk donors and developing methods for rapidly evaluating blood safety and transfusion practices.

HOW CDC AFFECTS POLICY

In addition to its formal recommendations and published policies, CDC influences policy regarding blood safety in a number of ways. One is the collection and publication of scientific data from studies such as those just described. Such data can have a significant impact, particularly when they are presented to venues such as the Blood Products Advisory Committee or when they become part of the CDC's congressional testimony or expert opinion to congressional staff. For example, largely on the basis of surveillance data on HIV type 2 (HIV-2) presented at the Blood Products Advisory Committee, FDA decided to defer HIV-2 screening until the HIV-1/HIV-2 combination screening enzyme immunoassay was licensed.

CDC also supports research in public health intervention, much of which directly affects transfusion medicine. For example, HIV counseling and testing sites were funded by CDC in 1985, partially to dissuade HIV-positive people from going to blood centers to be tested.

FORMAL RECOMMENDATIONS

There is no set formula for issuing formal recommendations, although there are some common steps. The first is to identify the problem. CDC has a national mandate to conduct infectious disease surveillance. State and local health departments and other agencies report unusual disease occurrences, particularly those that involve multiple states. Thus, CDC can rapidly identify large or unusual public health problems and, if appropriate, conduct an epidemiological study. One recent blood-related example was the matter of idiopathic $CD4^+$ T-lymphocytopenia (ICL). Once the potential problem was identified, CDC acted as a convener of transfusion experts and other relevant scientists to discuss it and implemented a surveillance system.

Occasionally, CDC will create interagency task forces within the public health service, such as the AIDS Executive Task Force which coordinated many of the early AIDS activities. These groups can then act as the sites for policy formulation.

Once the relevant information is gathered, recommendations are issued in draft form. CDC then tries to achieve consensus on the draft recommendations by, for example, hosting a meeting of experts and other relevant parties. A draft copy of the consensus is often sent to various constituency groups, and the draft recommendations are published in the *Federal Register*, particularly if the issue is one with a high profile. Public meetings may be held to discuss the issue further. A final recommendation may then be made and may be published in *MMWR* or in a scientific article. (The advantage of *MMWR* is that CDC can disseminate the recommendation and background information within 2 days.) The recommendations concerning donor screening made and published in *MMWR* prior to 1985 were formal recommendations by the U.S. Public Health Service, although notice was given that there was not a full consensus about them.

Other recommendations have addressed HIV antibody testing of blood and plasma, including topics such as interpretive criteria for Western blots, recommendations for screening, and what to tell and what not to tell a person who has been tested. Other recommendations concerning phlebotomy and laboratory procedures have been issued, such as universal precautions.

Blood Banking's Policy Groups and Procedures

Toby Simon

THE TRADITION OF SELF-REGULATION

It may be interesting to note that the American Board of Pathology is the only test committee that writes questions on regulations. The relationship between blood banking-transfusion medicine and government regulation is quite clear. It is understood that people seeking certification would know what was in the Code of Federal Regulation (CFR) and in the American Association of Blood Banks (AABB) standards. That does not happen elsewhere. Blood bankers are unusual among clinical pathologists, and laboratory medicine professionals in their interest in and involvement with regulations and standards. The regulatory context is inherent to what we do.

It is equally interesting to recall how amazed many people in blood banking were in 1972 when regulatory authority was transferred from the Division of Biologic Standards (more or less a part of the National Institutes of Health [NIH]) to the Food and Drug Administration (FDA). The tradition until then had been strongly one of *self*-regulation. Even with increased government involvement, self-regulation continues as a major theme today.

STANDARD-SETTING ORGANIZATIONS

A number of organizations are involved in self-regulation: The American Association of Blood Banks (AABB), the Council of Community Blood Centers (CCBC), the American Red Cross, and, with a lesser role, the College of American Pathologists. The American Blood Resources Association (ABRA) acts similarly with respect to plasma.

Each of these organizations has a role, although in standard setting AABB is the most active. The American Red Cross blood centers are not members of CCBC, yet because of its size, when the American Red Cross issues its blood service directives, they presumably affect some 45 to 50 percent of all operating blood centers and about half of the blood drawn and processed in the United States. That high percentage tends to create what lawyers would call a "standard of care." Thus, all blood centers must at least be aware of what the Red Cross is doing.

The College of American Pathologists conducts both a laboratory accreditation program and a survey program. Although most blood centers are not accredited by the college, many do use these surveys for purposes of the Clinical Laboratory Improvement Act (CLIA) regulation.

AMERICAN ASSOCIATION OF BLOOD BANKS

AABB is a volunteer organization with a board of trustees; a mixture of committed, well-trained volunteers who are active in the field and a growing professional staff; and various committees that deal with issues of importance. The Transfusion-Transmitted Diseases Committee, for example, assumed great importance in 1983 with the beginning of the AIDS epidemic.

The AABB has three different types of institutional members: blood centers that collect, manufacture, process, and distribute blood; hospital transfusion services that cross-match the units and distribute them to patients in a hospital; and a group, including some large hospitals, that do some of both. AABB also has over 8500 individual members from a wide variety of occupational settings, including the FDA.

The basis of AABB's self-regulation activity is the AABB standards. There is, in addition, the *Accreditation and Regulatory Manual*, called the ARM, which clarifies and interprets the standards. Inspection and accreditation procedures exist to ensure that the standards are being enforced.

A technical manual is also used by the organization to support its standard operating procedures. The technical manual is issued every 3 to 4 years so that new technical material is covered. The association also issues policies and recommendations to supplement the standards.

AABB publishes the scientific journal *Transfusion*. AABB also holds an annual meeting at which issues are raised, regulations can be discussed, and questions can be asked of AABB. FDA has recently participated in the question-and-answer programs. AABB also has various courses and educational materials that are important for the informed observance of the regulatory criteria.

The standards are published on an 18-month cycle; interim standards can also be issued as necessary. *The Standards* has a major advantage over CFR, in that it can be revised and published with some frequency and can be made readily available.

The self-regulatory and the government regulatory regimes are coordinated. AABB makes an effort not to be in conflict with FDA so that its members do not have to follow conflicting regulations. Thus, for example, *The Standards* incorporates guidelines and pronouncements of FDA that have not appeared in CFR. *The Standards*, although an instrument of voluntary regulation, incorporates government regulations and makes it available to the membership of the association in a user-friendly format. Moreover, *The Standards* seek to incorporate good medical practice and scientific data, wherever it is available, whether required by FDA regulations or not.

The standards-setting committee of AABB typically draws on the expertise of Centers for Disease Control and Prevention (CDC), FDA, the armed services, and others. Proposed standards are printed and circulated for comment before the recommended versions are sent to the Board of Directors for approval and invested with the imprimatur of the organization.

Members of AABB are expected to follow the standards to remain accredited. In alternate years AABB inspects each of its members. The inspection is done by volunteers or colleagues or by teams of volunteers and colleagues. When FDA's own enforcement activities increased, AABB noted that some members who had a very clean AABB inspection had problems only a few months later with an FDA inspection. It became obvious that AABB, using volunteers, could not put into its inspection activity the time and effort that an FDA investigator could when he or she was assigned to a facility for 2, 3, or 4 weeks or longer. In addition, AABB inspections tend to be collegial, contrast to the more obvious police-like aspects of an FDA visit.

AABB's first response was to try to use teams of inspectors for large, complex blood centers, with each member of a team having responsibility for one major area or department. That has worked to some extent, but it has still fallen short of providing for an AABB inspection what can be provided by FDA inspections. Thus, the direction most recently has been to emphasize a quality assurance program. AABB members should follow the program, and the main focus of AABB inspections is to make sure that they are doing so. AABB members are required to adopt a quality assurance plan that is based on the FDA Quality Assurance Guidelines, and the Association's own quality plan outline is available to guide members in this endeavor. The plan uses a system of self-assessment, documentation, correction and verification to ensure that facilities do not rely solely upon external auditors or inspectors to uncover problems.

JOINT EFFORTS

During the period of the emergence of the AIDS epidemic, AABB worked collaboratively in a number of areas with CCBC, the American Red Cross, and to some extent, ABRA. This has been the focus of some lawsuits that have described these efforts as conspiracies, which is a most unfortunate characterization. Surely if these organizations had *not* worked together the lawsuits would have claimed that each was irresponsible, going its own direction rather than working together to attack the problem.

Joint statements are no longer issued, but the four organizations still meet to discuss from time to time policy issues and to identify areas where they can work together and can engage in useful dialogue with FDA, CDC, and others in an effort to keep their activities moving in concert.

Typically, there will be a liaison from CCBC on the important committees of AABB, as there will be from the American Red Cross and, where appropriate, ABRA. CCBC's scientific/medical/technical committee frequently brings individuals from FDA to speak at its meetings, again, to ensure that there is effective dialogue.

OTHER STANDARDS AND GUIDELINES

In addition to AABB standards, the American Red Cross Blood Service Directives can be significant for other blood centers as well. ABRA, too, has recently developed a certification program—the Quality Plasma Program—to ensure that the manufacturers of source plasma adhere to a certain standard of quality. Generally, however, ABRA has not set standards. Plasma collection has a smaller number of standard operating procedures. Because plasma collection is dominated by larger manufacturers, with their responsibility for ensuring the quality of the source material, these firms' actions tend to be the origin of standards as they are approved by FDA. ABRA has had a formal FDA liaison committee for a number of years. This committee has been successful in improving the relationship between plasma collectors and regulators.

In 1989 or 1990 AABB followed suit and established such a committee for the blood collecting part of its activity. CCBC and the American Red Cross also participate, so that active liaison occurs from both the blood and the plasma portions of the blood banking community.

The College of American Pathologists (CAP) also conducts laboratory accreditation programs and surveys. These are of greater importance to hospitals than to blood banks. Almost all hospital transfusion services participate. For many years CAP has had deemed status with the Joint Commission on Accreditation of Healthcare Organizations for conducting the laboratory portion of hospital accreditation. CAP inspections therefore have great importance for hospitals that perform transfusion activity. CAP also conducts the surveys that are of great importance to CLIA certification, which blood banks also must have (until such time as FDA makes any changes). Like AABB, CAP uses volunteer inspectors, and like AABB, CAP has been having more trouble in recent years finding adequate numbers of volunteers to conduct the inspections.

Overall, self-regulating activity has certainly been an active area for blood banks. The emphasis is on adherence to standards and a regulatory mind-set on the part of the people who work in this field. The volunteer organizations believe that they do a good job of self-regulating and would like to emphasize that role and its importance as much as possible. It is an activity that has gone on more recently in concert with and in cooperation with federal regulatory activities to ensure that they are consistent.

Opportunities and Venues for Dialogue

Merlyn Sayers

THE CHANGING CLIMATE IN BLOOD BANKING

The climate within which alternative regulatory opportunities are being discussed has changed recently. The federal agencies that have an impact on decisions relating to blood safety are all agencies of the U.S. Public Health Service, and as such, they are headed by political appointees. Most political appointees are subject to the influence of those who appoint them.

Agency budgets largely depend on the goodwill of the members of the U.S. Congress. What is the character of that goodwill today? Republicans in the House of Representatives want a 6-month moratorium on federal regulatory activity. The Republican "Contract with America" included proposals to require federal agencies to go through an elaborate process not only of risk assessment but also of cost-benefit analysis before any future rules or regulations are promulgated. This is very different from what prevailed until even quite recently.

Other influences have also changed the climate in blood banking. There is a national blood shortage of alarming proportions. A recent American Red Cross press release reported severe shortages in 10 major cities, including Boston, Los Angeles, and Washington, D.C. The Red Cross reported that some 300,000 additional blood donations were required in the next month for the national inventory to be rendered safe.

The climate is also a little different on the legal front. Although litigation with regard to transfusion-transmitted AIDS may be in the eclipse, lawsuits are being brought elsewhere. In Australia, for example, individuals have brought lawsuits that have to do with the tardiness of the Australian Red Cross in introducing surrogate testing for non-A, non-B hepatitis. That retrospection may be visited upon U.S. blood programs in the not too distant future.

The Canadian Red Cross has recently undergone a painful and thorough outside review investigating inadequacies and inefficiencies in its performance. In the United States, the Food and Drug Administration (FDA) recently uncovered a whole range of flaws in the quality assurance programs of a major manufacturing company particularly with regard to the specificity of diagnostic products that are in wide use in blood programs. FDA believed that the rate of false-positive results in these diagnostic products was unacceptable, and because of the deficiencies found during FDA inspections, the agency has withheld approval of some of the company's newer diagnostic devices.

There are some bright lights, however. In January 1995 FDA held a public meeting to hear comments on the agency's regulations for blood products and establishments. The meeting is part of FDA Biologics Regulatory Review Project that started in June 1994 with the publication of documents reviewing general biologics and regulations for blood products and blood establishments. According to FDA, the purpose of the public hearing is to help the Center for Biologics Evaluation and Research to identify regulations that are "outdated, burdensome, inefficient or otherwise unsuitable or unnecessary in the interests of regulation.

VENUES FOR DIALOGUE

Opportunities for dialogue with FDA certainly exist. The process open to written public comment is flawed, as is anything that must move through the *Federal Register*. Even items that are a high priority can take 3 years to move through the system. That process is too lengthy for public influence to be of any real benefit.

The national blood banking organizations are themselves venues for dialogue. They have annual meetings, they have standards committees and scientific, medical, and technical committees, and they are platforms for dialogue between blood banking organizations and FDA. The American Association of Blood Banks (AABB) teleconferences are a good example. AABB organizes these teleconferences, linking as many as 80 or 90 blood banks around the country and discussing topics pertinent to blood banking.

THE BLOOD PRODUCTS ADVISORY COMMITTEE

FDA initiated advisory committee systems in the early 1970s to provide technical assistance related to the development and evaluation of drugs, biologics, and medical devices. The system was also designed to lend credibility to the agency's decisions and its decision-making processes. In addition, it was a means by which FDA could provide a forum for public discussions of controversial issues. In 1976 the Fountain Committee believed that the advisory committees might be too independent of FDA, and might be subject to the influence of drug sponsors. Curiously, by 1990 the concern was exactly the opposite. It was claimed by some that advisory committees were excessively influenced by FDA. In fact, however, the Blood Products Advisory Committee (BPAC) has always striven to be an independent source of information. Still, there was a perception that the BPAC's invited experts were under the heel of FDA. The high stakes associated with FDA decisions means that parties disappointed by the agency's action have strong incentives to charge that the independence of advisory committees is compromised by undue FDA influence.

Although incorrect, the criticism was nonetheless addressed in a number of ways. For one, FDA position papers that had been distributed to BPAC members in the past were discontinued, largely because, some suspected, a position paper would be evidence of the undue influence of FDA over the committee. The committee is also reminded that everything must be conducted in a fishbowl. There are no preliminary discussions among committee members and FDA. There is no discussion among committee members themselves prior to BPAC meetings. This has left the committee on some occasions a little uncertain as to exactly what the issues are, what FDA's position is, and in what area FDA best needs advice. BPAC has now maintained an unblemished reputation, although it may have been earned at the expense of the Committee's being able to give good and sound advice to FDA.

Although the advice of the advisory committee is not binding on FDA, its recommendations are widely regarded as a predictor of agency action. As a result, FDA advisory committees have become highly visible to the public, the U.S. Congress, and to the media. Some of the issues considered by BPAC in recent years include the following:

1. Yersinia.
2. Combination tests for HIV-1 and HIV-2.
3. Reducing red blood cell shelf-life.
4. Lookback for human T-lymphotropic leukemia virus types 1 and 2.
5. Recombinant factor VIII.
6. Use of "fresh" blood.
7. RIBA and reentry procedures.
8. Internal controls for antibody screening tests.
9. Bacterial contamination of platelets.
10. Idiopathic CD4 lymphocytopenia syndrome.
11. Postdonation "call back."
12. Hepatitis C virus testing relative to screening of plasma for fractionation.

OTHER VENUES FOR DIALOGUE

Other venues for dialogue include events such as single topic conferences. "Closing the HIV Window" was one recent conference topic. Private-sector conferences are also conducted, although they are sometimes sponsored by manufacturers who have an assay to promote or a product that they want to popularize. Thus, not all conferences are scientific in the fully unbiased sense.

The Institute of Medicine forums and the regional blood banking organizations may also be included as other venues for dialogue. Likewise, meetings of other national organizations like the Hemophilia Foundation, College of American Pathologists, the American Society for Apheresis, and the American Society of Hematology may also be opportunities for dialogue among scientists, blood bankers, and regulators.

In addition, alternative venues exist. The media is one of those venues, but good news does not earn Pulitzer Prizes. Bad news carries more credibility. The courts of law are venues as well. Most states regard blood as unavoidably unsafe, but blood programs are still vulnerable when it comes to acts of negligence. Hosts of lawsuits related to cases of transfusion-transmitted AIDS have been filed. The result of some of these have been that blood programs have added to their standard operating procedures practice for which there may be very thin evidence but which are done to avoid the risk of litigation.

THE VOICE OF BLOOD PRODUCT CONSUMERS

One of the criticisms of BPAC has come in the form that the committee represents a gang of cronies. Members of Congress have asked, "Where are the consumers on this committee?" implying that if consumers were represented on the committee, the right decisions would be made.

Appointment to BPAC has not exempted its members from possibly requiring a transfusion, nor has it exempted their family members from running the risk of requiring medical interventions, oncology treatment, or coronary artery bypass surgery. It is a hollow criticism to say that the decisions do not reflect consumer input. Everyone on BPAC is, will be, has been, or could be a consumer of the products on which the committee is asked to cast its opinions.

Editor's Note: During a later discussion of this topic, Thomas Zuck made the following point: "One difficulty is that we do not know who is going to be a blood recipient. One of four of us will be and some of us already have been. However, except for a few defined groups with hereditary diseases such as hemophilia, the rest are simply not known in advance. The American Blood

OVERVIEW OF REGULATION

Commission struggled with this issue of who can represent consumers, and we continue to struggle with it. But we are all consumers. It is folly to assume that we do not worry about consumers."

ATTENDING TO THE DONOR

The more important question is the more general one: "Who needs to be heard? Similarly, patients needing transfusions certainly need to be heard. Patients needing clotting factor concentrate need to be heard, as do blood bankers and manufacturers. The individuals at the cornerstone of blood banking practice and patient transfusion care nationally, however, not heard. These are the blood donors. Any regulatory revision must take into account this neglected group of individuals. Their support of blood programs is probably at the lowest level that it has ever been for reasons largely related to the effects of regulation, which in a number of different areas penalizes them. They are now subjected to a level of scrutiny that none would have expected 5 or 10 years ago. They are subjected to questioning that is nothing short of an Inquisition. They are subjected to an increasing number of tests. Not only are the tests non-specific, but so are the questions.

To see the effect of this nonspecificity on donations, consider what statisticians call "contours of constant probability of inappropriate deferral. The bottom axis of such a contour graph is the specificity of the screening test; on the vertical axis is the number of donations. If the tests have relatively high specificity, for example, 98 percent, an uninfected donor still has a 25 percent chance of deferral after 12 or so donations—that is, deferral for reasons of nonspecificity, not for reasons of true positives. If that test specificity decays down to about 95 percent, that same individual has a 25 percent chance of deferral after only five donations.

If those tests and questions were to decay in combination to a specificity of perhaps 50 percent, at that point the donor would have a 90 percent chance of deferral after only four donations. This system thus penalizes the very individual most valuable to the process, namely, the repeat volunteer donor.

REGULATORY DIFFICULTIES

Where are the problems in regulation today? Regulation is tardy. New regulation cannot keep pace with science, and the blood programs sense that regulation is applied inconsistently. Some blood programs have the impression that the attitude of compliance inspectors is sometimes one of disbelief and a suspicion that the blood programs have something to hide.

Discussion

It was observed during the Forum's discussions that one of the areas in which safety and risk are affected by standards and practice is the medical decision to transfuse blood. Inappropriate transfusion is, or at least adds to, the possibility of transfusion-transmitted disease. The Forum explored briefly how that aspect of the process is or is not regulated.

Richard Shapiro: One of the categories of people who should be involved in the discussion are the people who make the decision to transfuse—the physician. The problems of both undertransfusion and overtransfusion exist. Constraining transfusion to appropriate uses needs to be taken into account as well.

Toby Simon: AABB, which includes among its members scientists and physicians in various fields, has been developing guidelines for appropriate utilization. A number of programs going back to the mid-1980s have produced publications, teaching aids, and handbooks on the question, in addition to a number of conferences, lectures, and materials. The National Institutes of Health (NIH) has had a role in two ways. One is the consensus development conference, including some on plasma, platelet, and red blood cell transfusions that addressed the indications for transfusion in an attempt to reduce them to the needed number. NIH also conducted, again in concert with other organizations, the National Blood Resource Education Program. There were a number of activities for physicians, including educational materials.

It is clear that the most efficient way to prevent a transfusion complication is not to transfuse, but there has also been concern recently about undertransfusion. It is not clear where the balance is in the physician community between risking inappropriate transfusion and withholding a possibly beneficial transfusion. Both may be now occurring in substantial numbers.

Unidentified Participant: There are not many data with which to make solid recommendations about when to transfuse. Wide variations in the practice suggest that not everyone is doing it correctly, but we do not yet know enough. More research is needed in this area.

Toby Simon: Studies with humans are difficult to do and are usually open to methodological criticisms. They do not fare well in the peer review process, and it has been very difficult to get them funded.

Elaine Eyster: Many of the transfusions in this country are initiated by house officers, at least in teaching hospitals. Often, the attending physician does not find out about it until after the patient has received the transfusion. Perhaps there should be efforts to work with medical schools and training program directors to develop algorithms for given situations.

Thomas Zuck: Many medical schools face the problem of competition, particularly in the senior year—for educational time. Transfusion medicine must compete with everything else; it is extremely difficult to get the hours.

Toby Simon: The Transfusion Medicine Academic Awards was an NIH program supported by the AABB, CCBC, CAP and others that was carried out for a number of years. The literature describes the practice of the "just-in-time" consult, in which a physician expert in transfusion medicine is involved immediately on receiving an order. This could be very effective with house officers in particular. The College of American Pathologists does support the effort through its work in the Joint Commission, by their Requirement for Transfusion Committees and Review. But all of these have fallen short of what we want to achieve, however.

Arthur Caplan: In many hospitals the transfusion committees are now called "utilization and review committees." That is, a heavy emphasis is placed on guidelines for transfusion within hospitals. Active program utilization review is short of the ideal, but it does exist and is an ongoing activity. It may now be at the point at which most of the business of those committees is the review of transfusions given outside the guidelines. It is not a total vacuum in terms of utilization review and efforts to teach algorithms or standards.

Elaine Eyster: We must take the next steps. Transfusion information has not been well disseminated. Most teaching hospitals are not practicing those steps, and are not likely to find it possible to have a knowledgeable advisor available at the time of every transfusion.

II

Regulatory Enforcement and Compliance

CBER Compliance Activity

James Simmons

COORDINATION BETWEEN THE CENTERS AND THE FIELD

A question that blood bankers sometimes raise is that of inspectional consistency. To better understand that issue, we should begin with the basics of the interaction between Food and Drug Administration (FDA) headquarters and its operations in the field.

FDA has five product-specific centers—the centers for foods, drugs, devices, veterinary medicine and biologics—and one process-oriented unit, namely, the Office of the Associate Commissioner for Regulatory Affairs, all of which report to the Commissioner through the Deputy Commissioner for Operations. The Center for Biologics Evaluation Research (CBER) has the principal responsibility for the regulation of blood; the Associate Commissioner for Regulatory Affairs has the principal responsibility for establishing regulatory inspectional policies and procedures.

The product-related centers and the process-oriented Office of Regulatory Affairs interact at various levels. It is difficult to separate all of these functions clearly, but to a large extent, it can be said that the product-related centers have responsibility for scientific review of new product applications and the establishment of product standards, specifications, and regulations such as current good manufacturing practices (GMPs). The Associate Commissioner for Regulatory Affairs and his or her staff are responsible for enforcement policies and procedures and for inspectional activities for all five product-related centers.

Each of these organizations has subdivisions. Reporting to the Director of CBER are three product-related offices—blood, vaccines, and therapeutics—and some function-related offices such as the Office of Management, the Office of Establishment Licenses, and the Office of Compliance. These units within CBER service all three product-related CBER offices.

The Office of Compliance is responsible for providing compliance enforcement inspectional activities for the product-related offices. It bears the primary responsibility for establishing policies and guidance that go to the field inspection staff.

OFFICE OF REGULATORY AFFAIRS

The Office of Regulatory Affairs (ORA) also has various components with specialized functions. It includes all of the field personnel, who report directly to the Associate Commissioner for Regulatory Affairs through the six regional directors and other field structures. Also in that office are support offices to the field, one of which is the Office of Regional Operations, which is responsible for providing direction, guidance, and support to the field, and in providing such services, it ensures inspectional uniformity.

There is a good deal of coordination between the Office of Compliance at CBER and the Office of Regional Operations at ORA, including a number of shared responsibilities; for example, the offices jointly develop good manufacturing practices (GMP) regulations, inspectional guides, procedural manuals, and training programs. In the development of these programs, each office takes the responsibility for soliciting input from its respective organizations and for disseminating output to the same organizations.

The inspections are coordinated in accordance with guides developed by this process. The reports of violations that may proceed from these inspections come back from the field offices to the Office of Compliance and to CBER for review. After receipt, they are evaluated and decisions are made concerning the appropriate regulatory or enforcement action, if such action is indicated.

That is a rather highly condensed review of the nature of the headquarters-field interaction, but it leads to a few observations about the question of inspectional consistency.

INSPECTION CONSISTENCY

It is important that we clearly define the issues and understand the magnitude of the problem. Although there is much debate about uniformity of inspections, there may be some confusion regarding the relationship between inspectional uniformity and enforcement uniformity. Yet another term, "regulatory uniformity," has an even broader connotation. The term "inspections" is more focused; it describes a site visit at a regulated establishment for the purpose of determining compliance with laws and regulations.

Inspections may be comprehensive, covering all phases of the operation, or they may be limited to one or a few regulated activities. For example, limited inspections are frequently conducted as part of a follow-up to complaints, product recalls, or adverse experience reports. They would concentrate on the specific area of concern and not on all activities of the establishment. Some critics who point to inconsistencies of inspections fail to take into consideration the impacts of the different types of inspections. It would be inappropriate to expect a limited inspection to reveal the same findings as a comprehensive inspection. That is one of the factors that is not always taken into consideration when one suggests that there is a high degree of nonuniformity or a lack of consistency in the inspection process.

INSPECTIONS AND ENFORCEMENT

The word "enforcement" refers not to an inspection but rather to the administrative or legal sanctions taken in response to documented long-standing or serious violations. Although an inspection usually precedes an enforcement action, not all inspections result in enforcement actions. In fact, only 5 to 10 percent of all inspections lead to enforcement of any sort, and the enforcements themselves range from serious penalties like injunctions or license suspensions down to the simple and much more common issuance of a letter of warning.

The statute provides for a range of enforcement actions, with each one having a clearly defined objective. Some are meant to stop the further distribution of violative products already in distribution channels; others are meant to remedy the conditions that may cause violations before additional products are produced. The choice of one enforcement action over another requires a consideration of the nature and severity of the problem, its frequency of occurrence and its duration, past efforts to remedy the problem, the distribution status of products, the establishment's compliance history, and a number of other factors. It is clearly appropriate to take different enforcement actions in response to different inspections even if the inspectional findings themselves are nearly identical.

The decisions to take different enforcement actions in the presence of similar inspectional findings may lead to the appearance of inconsistency. Neither a uniform process for conducting inspections nor a uniform process for enforcement decision-making, however, will produce uniform results unless there is uniformity of operations that are subject to the inspection. Those of us who see uniformity do so on the basis of uniformity of the process. Those who see nonuniformity do so on the basis of the results of the process. As we examine this issue of inspectional consistency, we need to make sure that we are distinguishing between the process and the results of the process.

FDA Practice in the Field

Richard Swanson

TRAINING FOR THE FIELD

FDA has about 1,040 investigators spread throughout the United States in six regions, 21 district offices, and 135 resident posts. About 350 of FDA's 1,040 investigators have had national training in the inspectional activities of blood and blood products. Two national experts and three regional experts are involved in the inspectional activities of blood and blood products. Because industry has not remained stagnant over the years, training is not a one-time effort. Therefore, continuous training is required.

Training contributes to consistency, as do FDA's guides and regulations. Industry has access to those guides and to the training manuals and inspectors' operational manuals. These can be used to see how we are going to do an inspection and whether we have quality assurance within those situations to ensure consistency with inspectional observations.

SOURCES OF CONSISTENCY

The basis of consistency begins with the *Code of Federal Regulations*. FDA has, in addition, a regulatory procedures manual that describes how it establishes the regulatory posture on a particular item, such as blood and blood products. The compliance policy guides on biologics are spelled out in another manual.

The words in the manuals mean the same to each of those 350 investigators. The investigators, however, are not robots who see everything in exactly the same way. Investigators see the same set of facts in various ways, leading to various interpretations. To expect that every one of 350 people is going to have exactly the same observation is unrealistic, yet we do have enough supervisory review to pick out any outliers. This would be a quality assurance process in itself.

An additional guidance is the investigations operational manual, which spells out the specific parameters that the inspector should to look for and examine further in an inspection. FDA has gone further, by publishing a guide to the inspection of blood banks, conducting training sessions with industry, having grassroots seminars with industry, and producing materials for industry and health professionals. On this basis FDA is attempting to ensure uniformity and consistency.

FDA has expanded our dialogues with the industry. FDA's Field Biologic Committee has had numerous opportunities to talk with segments of the industry through trade associations. As we start seeing a dynamic change in the government in the next 5 years with the downsizing and with the flattening of government, with the restriction of resources, it is going to behoove us all to make sure that consistency remains.

In the past few years we have had annual inspections of blood banks. That has now been reduced to looking at the compliance of various firms. The firms that are in compliance are inspected every other year. We are still inspecting 100 percent of plasma facilities yearly, however, things do change, and these things have improved.

Challenges and Questions About Compliance

William Sherwood

Current compliance procedures are subject to a number of challenges. Although they are most frequently questions without obvious answers, it will nonetheless be important to answer some of these questions in the coming months and years.

IMPROVEMENTS IN SAFETY

During the past 12 to 15 years there has been an enormous improvement in the safety of the blood supply and this is an accepted fact. Blood transfusions are not 100 percent safe, but we are almost at a position of *de minimis* risk. Many studies and examples demonstrate that improvement in safety. One particular example, however, does provide an interesting additional feature of the safety of the blood supply. The data are from case reports of clinical transfusion-associated hepatitis reported to the American Red Cross blood service region in Philadelphia over a 10-year period beginning in 1981. There had been an active reporting mechanism during that period to seek out such cases at the hospital level and to report them to the Blood Center to identify donors that should be deferred. These cases of *clinical* transfusion-associated hepatitis are only the tip of the hepatitis iceberg, but we can assume that, like an iceberg, what is found at the tip is proportional to what is found at the bottom.

The data provided the number of cases of transfusion-associated hepatitis over 6-month intervals. Consider just two points: in 1981 there were 75 reports. In 1991, there were two. During the 10-year period from 1981 to 1991, the Blood Center increased it collections from 290,000 to 360,000 units, or about 100,000 additional components at risk. Through 1995, with the same system still in place, we are still experiencing only one, two, or three reports of hepatitis a year.

I believe that these data illustrate another phenomenon. Surrogate testing for non-A, non-B hepatitis (alanine aminotransferase and hepatitis B core antibody testing) was initiated in 1985 and 1986; anti-hepatitis C virus (anti-HCV) testing was initiated in 1991; and although there could be a debate about the effectiveness of the deferral of high-risk groups, the introduction of surrogate and anti-HCV testing had a profound effect on clinical transfusion-associated hepatitis. The correlations with the data intervals seem apparent; this point should be kept in mind as we proceed.

QUESTIONS ABOUT ENFORCEMENT

Four basic questions need to be raised. The first question is quite direct:

Are the current regulatory compliance methods, techniques, and institutions the best approach to ensuring the safest and most effective blood supply possible for the American people?

This question may seem irreverent at best, considering the acts of Congress that established Food and Drug Administration (FDA) and that conveyed authority to it, the success that FDA has experienced over the years, and the reverence that the agency enjoys throughout the world. As we look for ways to improve, however, the very basis of our institutions sometimes needs to change in order to make progress. Some areas clearly seem to need fixing, yet there have been few regulatory changes in recent years. This may be the result of a cumbersome regulatory process. The agency has resorted to publishing guidelines that have the effect of regulation to keep up with our dynamic environment. The licensing process is interminably slow. I suspect that is a resource problem for the agency, but the question is still a broad one, and one that needs to be proposed.

Evidence That Compliance Works

The second of the four questions is as follows:

Is there evidence that the current approach, of law, regulation, inspection, observation and sanction is effective?

The key word in this question is "evidence." There is clearly good evidence that the general policies intended to improve blood safety such as the introduction of donor deferral policies and serologic testing have been very successful. Much of the credit for those tests has a basis in FDA and its regulation. This question, however, is intended to deal with the compliance process as well.

What is the incremental contribution to blood safety that the compliance process adds? Can we point to evidence of results from the compliance process that benefit the public?

Perhaps it is unfair to separate the rule-making and the licensing processes from the compliance process and to give each the burden of providing proof of its effectiveness. The current paradigm of law and regulation must include a process for enforcement. That much is accepted. A technical and scientific world however, requires data to demonstrate effectiveness, which in this case is not the gross weight of Form 483 (post inspection reports of noncompliance) and the number of observations, but more the prevention of disease and the improved quality of products and services. That is what we would be looking for. Maybe the relevance of the question is itself an issue: regardless of the data, FDA could rightly argue that it has the responsibility to uphold the law, whether there is an effectiveness to its methods that can be demonstrated or not.

This point leads to the third question:

Is there such evidence of effectiveness for the compliance process? If there is, are the outcomes that benefit the American people proportionate and consistent with the effort expended by both government and industry?

Useful data on effectiveness about an isolated compliance process would be difficult to obtain. There are many variables, and there are likely both direct and indirect effects. The direct effects follow from the inspections themselves, along with the observations on Form 483 and the corrective actions that are taken as a result of those observations. However, there are also indirect effects.

Indirect Effects: "Bulletproofing"

The behaviors that blood establishments undertake in attempts to "bulletproof" themselves against future FDA inspections, may well be the behavior that has the greatest practical impact, so deserves some additional scrutiny.

In my experience, FDA inspections have been variable and uneven. It is not unusual for an establishment to receive a number of annual inspections, receive no Form 483s or receive little in the way of observations, and then suddenly to be totally surprised and receive a devastating inspection, with multiple pages of Form 483 and perhaps worse. Changes in the performance of blood establishments, occur over time, but those changes do not have the same degree of variability seen with FDA inspections. This circumstance creates a behavior in blood centers by which systems and procedures may be put in place to provide some armor for the blood center against the worst case scenario: the most aggressive FDA inspection and, in particular, the widest possible interpretation of the regulations. The establishments thus find themselves invoking systems and procedures that they believe do not contribute to the safety, purity, or efficacy of the blood supply. These actions may not be required by a narrow interpretation of the regulations, but they are put in place in anticipation of the worst-case possibility. This behavior carried to an extreme has many consequences. Blood centers lose sight of what is important. It is a drain on resources, people, and money, that otherwise could be directed to research and development, to new products and services, and to meaningful improvements in quality.

Today, blood establishments cannot afford to do anything that is not important. Most blood centers are not-for-profit, have little or no reserves, and are in a poor position to increase their revenues through the health care system. Unlike some firms in the for-profit pharmaceutical industry, they cannot afford to have a legion of quality assurance staff.

Blood establishments rely heavily on operational staff to perform double duty in procedure development, training, and quality control. In other words, government spends an enormous sum to ensure compliance, and industry spends multiples of that to carry it out. The public pays for it at both ends. Is the public getting its money's worth in the process?

Is Compliance Improving?

The fourth question is as follows:

Is our industry improving in its compliance behavior and if not, why?

Here is a troubling observation: In the early 1980s, at about the time that it became clear that the human immunodeficiency virus (HIV) could be transmitted by blood, FDA focused attention on the blood industry, as well it should have. The industry has now enjoyed at least 12 years of this attention. The safety of the blood supply today is enormously improved over what it was 12 years ago, but what is the regulatory record of the industry now at the end of these 12 years? The largest blood collection organization is under a consent decree. The next largest one has received an intent-to-close notice. At least one of the largest independent centers has received a serious warning letter. It is a simple fact that a large proportion of the blood collected in the United States is under significant regulatory sanction.

Is it true that although the safety of the blood supply has improved, the regulatory performance of the industry has worsened? As the earlier question posed, are blood safety and regulatory performance unlinked, or are we dealing with a timing issue—a frameshift problem in terms of blocks of time and improvements in safety and regulatory matters? If we are not improving and if after 12 years of trying we continue to worsen, why is that so? Is it an industry problem? Haven't we "gotten it" yet? Is it an agency problem? Or is it both? If we continue on the same course, should we be looking forward to a time when the blood supply will have reached an ultimate degree of safety, yet our regulatory performance will have worsened to the degree that there will not be any qualified blood centers to distribute it? That is, of course, hyperbole to make the point. Clearly, we hope that our safety improves, and we hope that our compliance performance improves as well.

REGULATION AND OTHER FORCES

There is a much that moves us to try to do the right thing, only one factor of which is the regulatory apparatus. Beyond that are our own concerns with quality assurance. The mission statements of many blood banking organizations are such that we are not carrying out our job if we are not doing it in a way that meets the needs of and benefits the people. Our people intend to be honest in that way. There is in also the specter of tort litigation. In the United States that is a profound aspect, and we do a great deal because of it. If we are in violation of the law, whether we receive a Form 483 on it or not, if we are inspected or not, if it causes harm to a patient we are in trouble. Thus, although there is a role for regulation, compliance, and enforcement, that is not the only thing that moves us to do the right thing.

Discussion

Question from the Audience: Language conveys meaning. Why are Food and Drug Administration (FDA) enforcement people called "investigators" rather than "inspectors"? These titles have very different meanings. The fire inspector comes around to look at your place and see if everything is all right, but the fire investigator comes to examine whether a fire should be called arson. The feeling of these things is important. They set a stage of cooperation and noncooperation.

Richard Swanson: It might be confusing to you, but we also have a group of people called inspectors. There are about 150 people who have the title inspector. This question points out the need for us to have a dialogue with each other so that we understand our nomenclature, understand how we can talk, and, understand the difference between an inspector and an investigator and a compliance officer.

Question from the Audience: Are the contents of the various manuals and booklets that you described regulations or guidelines or both, and how are changes distributed and explained?

James Simmons: In the last several months, if not longer, there has been a debate about the difference between regulations and guidelines. The charge has been made that FDA in particular is issuing guidelines but is trying to enforce them as regulations, and that the investigators have been trying to take the guidelines and act as if they were law.

There is a debate even among legal scholars about some of these distinctions, but for our purposes, these manuals are meant to provide guidance to the inspectors, telling them how to do their job. Since all of this information is available to the public, some people choose to call them guidelines. Certainly, that sort of document does not rise to the level of being a formal regulation. Most of them are intended to be procedural guides and instructions—not that different, perhaps, from the industry's own use of standard operating procedures. They tell the inspectors how to present their credentials and how to issue a notice of inspection, how to write a Form 483, who to talk with at the conclusion of the inspection, and other things of that sort. All of these internal documents are updated periodically, sometimes as much as annually and possibly even more often.

Richard Swanson: *The Code of Federal Regulations (CFR)* contains the regulations that we are asked to enforce. All of the other documents are procedures designed to provide consistency, to guide inspectors, and to have the industry be able to be prepared for what we expect.

James Simmons: It is interesting to speculate about what would happen if these documents were not out there. If you just handed the basic statute that was passed by Congress to 500 different individuals and let them make their own interpretations of what it meant, we would have far more non-uniformity than is perceived to be there now. All of these other documents are designed to assure greater uniformity, though it sometimes seems from the dialogue that it is perceived to be quite the opposite.

Richard Swanson: The regulatory procedures manual and the investigator's operational manual go through a clearance process and a review by our General Counsel, so that the legal interpretation is also subjected to review.

Question from the Audience: How would you answer the question of whether there is any evidence that the system of law, regulation, inspection, compliance, and sanction is effective? Has the Office of Compliance done any cost-effectiveness studies of its own regulatory activities? Is there, on the other hand, evidence of reactions similar to the wasteful practice of "defensive medicine"?

James Simmons: The rate of compliance in 1993 was about 93 percent. That means that 7 percent of the inspections concluded that a firm was out of compliance to the point that enforcement action would be appropriate. In 1994 that dropped to about 5 percent. At present, data for 10 months of 1995 are available and that figure is about 3 percent. I believe that the total degree of compliance in the blood industry is higher than most people expect it to be.

Dramatic improvements have been made in the state of compliance. It takes some time to turn around big organizations that have widespread noncompliance, but once these things start falling in place, they make tremendous improvements, and I have personally observed many improvements in the area of compliance. Therefore, improvements in compliance are occurring. There is a presumption that the regulations lead to safety.

As to the cost-effectiveness, the only studies done at FDA are those examining the costs of our own operations. We have almost no method of doing industry costs. In proposing new regulations, there is an economic impact statement, but we do not have the capabilities for doing the kind of cost-effectiveness study that you described.

The tendency to build a "fire wall" to prevent future Form 483 observations is a critical point that needs to be made. I suspect that some people in all of the industries that FDA regulates go beyond what would be necessary to correct the problem, and if anybody is involved in that process, I would firmly recommend that you consult with the agency in terms of correcting your remedies.

Question from the Audience: FDA published its last inspection checklists book in 1991. The checklists were used by the blood banks and donor centers to identify which parts of the CFR or which memorandum or guidance was being applied in a 483. That check-off list has been eliminated, allowing the inspectors—who are mostly not blood bankers—to apply anything they are comfortable with. Now when one asks the inspector, "Can you please identify which CFR or memoranda that 483 is against?" they reply that legal counsel has told them they cannot identify it.

James Simmons: We should start with the culture of FDA and its inspection staff. As you know, blood establishments were not subject to FDA inspections until 1972, yet this agency had a history of almost 70 years of inspectional procedures prior to the time it started inspecting blood establishments. The traditional FDA units have never used a checklist. In 1972, when we started inspecting blood establishments, because it was such a new area the management of the agency thought it would be helpful to have such a checklist. Blood establishment inspections were not the only ones for which a list was used. Responsibility for regulating blood and blood products came to FDA from existing U.S. Public Health Service agencies in the 1960s and early 1970s, along with the Radiological Health Program, the Interstate Milk Shippers' Program, and a program that dealt with sanitation of interstate carriers like buses, trains, and airplanes. All of those programs, and several others, which were traditional Public Health Service programs when they were brought into FDA, brought checklist type forms, and for the most part, employees who were formerly with the Public Health Service units that did that work came to FDA. They were familiar with the form. They transferred with the transfer of functions and they continued using the form, even though the traditional FDA inspectors had never used checklists, and quite frankly, we had difficulties getting them to accept a checklist. Traditional thought in FDA is that checklists put blinders on the inspectors, in that they look at certain things and are not able to look at the broader spectrum. As a result of these kinds of discussions the agency did away with the checklist but left it as an option for inspectors to use if they chose to do so.

Inspectors should probably not have to list *CFR* citations. One of the reasons why the Office of General Counsel does not like the concept is that investigators are not attorneys; they do not want them to give an incorrect citation. We have even eliminated the requirement of putting *CFR* citations in our warning letters. The concept is simply to tell the establishment in lay terms what is perceived to be wrong and to let them make the corrections. If you look at the statutory intent of the Form 483, it is to be a communication device from the inspector to the establishment. It is not meant for third parties. It merely says, on the part of the inspector, that "during the course of my inspection I observed the following conditions which may lead to adulterated products." It does not say that the product is adulterated. It is intended to identify things that may cause adulteration if they are not corrected. Some of those things may not necessarily be that applicable to a *CFR* citations, as opposed to being a helpful tool. Unfortunately, we have gotten to the point in our relationships between inspectors and establishments that sometimes it does not look like a helpful tool.

Question from the Audience: How are the guidelines that come from the agency and that are intended for the inspectors developed, and how can the blood banking establishments provide feedback to that process?

James Simmons: If it is a technical or a scientific matter, the policy largely comes from work done within the Office of Blood, and the Office of Compliance and the Center for Biologics Evaluation and Research (CBER). We then incorporate the feedback from the Office of Regional Operations. If the issue relates to procedures, it usually emanates from the Office of Regional Operations. We have a system that is not dissimilar from that of the Blood Products Advisory Committee, which the agency uses to elicit feedback from the regulated industries and scientific experts within FDA. Twice a year we have an advisory committee meeting between CBER and some of the field managers who have identified problem areas and who have asked for guidance. Once the guidance is requested, we start the process of obtaining input from the Office of Blood and from the Office of Compliance. In consultation with the Office of Regional Operations, we try to develop the process. Unfortunately, we get many more requests than we can fulfill because we simply do not have enough time to answer all of the procedural requests.

What is ironic is that the more of these requests that we receive and the more specific the guidance that we give out, the more they become seen as regulations. We are then told that we are overregulating, yet if we try not to answer one of the questions, whether it is a request from industry or from one of our field staff, we are on the other side of the dilemma. Either we provide the guidance or we do not, and we get criticized on both points. I do not have an answer to that dilemma.

Question from the Audience: At present what may be found to provoke an enforcement action in New York may not be an enforcement action in Cincinnati, or vice versa. Do you perceive this change?

James Simmons: Because there is great criticism throughout the country about our inspections, there has been an effort to bring about some kind of change. The management of FDA and some of the people who advocate change have not clearly defined what that change should be. Although everybody recognizes that we could make some improvements in some areas, there is a role for an inspector in the changing environment. I am not sure that the role is going to change. I think that the methods and procedures for doing business will change, but I think that the role is pretty well fixed.

Question from the Audience: Just as the data show improvements in blood safety, there has also been an improvements in the quality of automobiles. The methodology that got us there have not been the same, however. There are approaches to safety other than the one now used at FDA. Total quality management, for example, is a very different approach. It is not a punitive regulatory approach nearly as much as it is achieving the highest possible quality through positive incentives.

James Simmons: We are looking at the regulatory procedures used by other agencies and these show some things might be done differently. There is, for example, much interest in third-party certification. We have operated with the same regulatory process for almost 100 years and although I cannot see that we are ever going to do away with regulations, the methods of approaching them could be different, and your suggestions would be helpful.

Perhaps the culture that we are talking about has some relationship to past and present organizational changes and responsibilities. The former Center for Biologics was a very strong science-based organization. Most of the people there did a little bit of everything, including research, investigational new drug applications, review, inspection, standard writing, and just about the whole potpourri of what goes on in the current CBER. The inspectors in the field were in constant touch with the science-based policy that was developing from day to day. My sense is that starting in 1972, when FDA took over that responsibility, the field inspections drifted away from CBER. The FDA field offices ares now more in charge of inspections. The interface between the field offices with CBER may be less than what it has been. If that interface were closer, perhaps we would see less of the difficulty of inspectors operating in a vacuum, more so than they did years ago. They would have more of a science-based tradition behind them. Compliance and science would be joining science-based tradition behind them. Compliance and science would be joining hands better, and the regulated industry would find it more palatable.

We are not all the way to the point that you have described, because in fact, the only part of CBER inspections done in the field environment is blood and blood product inspections; and now that is limited primarily to the annual inspections, not the preapproval inspections. Interestingly, however, the primary motivation for doing that was itself uniformity. This shows how we sometimes chase ourselves around in a circle.

Richard Swanson: The organizational chart presents only a part of the picture. Communications occur not only through solid and dotted lines. The Field Biological Committee has an interface across many avenues. Enforcement and inspection must be a team effort, and so the formal lines are interconnected with additional communications.

III

Innovations and Alternatives in Regulation

Regulatory Alternatives

Sidney Shapiro

In 1982, U.S. Supreme Court Justice Stephen Breyer, who was then a professor of law at the Harvard Law School, suggested a metaphor to describe regulatory reform. He proposed that regulatory failure should be understood as an issue of match and mismatch. According to Breyer, a regulatory failure occurs when government fails to match correctly the problem and the regulatory tool.

A mismatch can occur for either of two reasons. First, government can misdiagnose the problem that it is attempting to solve and therefore apply the wrong regulatory approach. For example, it is now widely recognized that government regulation of transportation markets was based on the erroneous perception that unrestrained competition would result in monopolization.

Second, even if the problem is correctly identified, regulatory tools vary in their effectiveness and cost. A partial mismatch occurs when government relies on a regulatory tool that is less effective or more expensive than another option would have been.

REGULATORY DIAGNOSIS AND MISMATCH

Critics of regulation argue that the failure to balance the costs and benefits of health and safety regulation has burdened economic development and wasted scarce resources. The Delaney Clause is the most prominent example of this criticism. It requires Food and Drug Administration (FDA) to ban the use of any food additive that causes cancer in laboratory animals, even if there is only a *de minimis* risk to humans.

A related problem is the government's attempt to remove what Breyer calls "the last 10 percent of a risk." Breyer notes that it is often so expensive to buy this extra margin of safety that the cost of doing so is likely to exceed the benefits to be gained. In such cases the country might be better off with more modest attempts at reducing health and safety risks: because of the high cost of excess risk reduction, critics point out that less money is available to address more significant risks. For example, it would be far less expensive, and perhaps no less safe, to fence off some Superfund sites instead of cleaning them up to the point where someone can eat the dirt with little or no risk.

In summary, the reformers are critical of policy choices that cannot be reconciled with cost-benefit analysis. They object to spending more money to reduce a risk than the economic benefits that are gained from reducing it.

However, other policy analysts respond that citizens may use a non-economic yardstick when they decide what level of risk is appropriate. We need not presume or deny that consumer attitudes are "irrational" or "unscientific" or that individual citizens necessarily misperceive the actual probabilities of risk. This is a different point. Assume that consumers adequately understand the probabilities of risk, but that they object to quantifying or comparing the costs and benefits of those risks. Citizens may choose certain risk policies, for example, because they promote such values as individual autonomy or fairness rather than a balancing of risks and benefits.

As the philosopher Carl Cranor notes, citizens may decide that some things are more important than producing net community benefits. If risk policies are to serve both economic and non-economic goals, regulators face difficult questions concerning the trade-offs. Mark Sagoff, also a philosopher, has written concerning environmental law: "The role of the policy maker and of the legislature may be to balance what we believe in and stand for as a community with what we want and need as a functioning economy. The future of environmental policy rests on facilitating the balance of interests with morality and one morality with another morality." This is no easy job.

Thus, the choice of the appropriate regulatory goal is confounded by the definition of the regulatory problem. The definition of risk as an economic problem produces one diagnosis, whereas the definition of risk as a problem of other social values produces another.

MAXIMIZING EFFECTIVENESS AND EFFICIENCY

Even after the problem is defined, there remains the question of which regulatory option is the most appropriate. As Justice Breyer has indicated, a partial mismatch occurs when the government relies on a regulatory tool that is less effective and more expensive than an alternative.

According to many critics, a significant source of regulatory failure is the use of rigid, highly bureaucratic command-and-control regulations. In command and control regulation, government specifies the method of compliance that a regulated entity is to use. For example, the regulation of air, water and workplace conditions relies on the use of the "best available technology"; that is, all firms are required to act to the level of the best available technology to reduce a particular risk. Another example is FDA requiring drug manufacturers to adopt a particular method to ensure the sterility of a product.

Critics have made three general criticisms of command-and-control regulation. The first is an efficiency-based criticism, that is, that command-and-control approaches are inefficient in terms of society's resources. They are also expensive because uniform standards ignore diversity among firms' abatement costs and because they may not permit the regulated entities to adopt new technologies that are equally effective and less costly.

A second criticism relates to innovation. Command-and-control regulations discourage research and innovation concerning new regulatory technology if they do not permit the adoption of such technology.

Finally, command-and-control regulations encourage strong political opposition because they are inefficient and discourage innovation. By comparison, the critics assert, less stringent—that is, more reasonable—regulation would be easier to adapt and adopt because there would be less opposition. Thus, critics of command-and-control contend that it is inefficient, that it discourages innovation, and that it encourages regulatory opposition.

These charges are true, no doubt, to some extent but they also overstate for several reasons the failure of the existing systems. First, the implementation of command-and-control schemes tends to take into account intraindustry and other differences that affect efficiency. Agencies typically use variances and other devices to account for these differences. Secondly, agencies more often tend to use efficient systems of command-and-control than inefficient systems. Finally, some research has indicated that regulatory entities tend to oppose less stringent regulatory initiatives with the same vigor as they oppose stricter proposals. The reason is simple: delay typically saves regulated entities money, and given enough time, the political environment could change in favor of the regulatory entity.

Nonetheless, reformers urge three kinds of reforms of command-and-control: more flexible regulations, market-based incentives, and voluntary approaches. It is important, first, to note that command-and-control regulations also come in three flavors. A command-and-control regulation can be a specification standard, a design standard, or a performance standard. A specification standard is one that specifies a particular technology to be used. For example, the U.S. Congress has directed that new hazardous waste landfills and surface impoundments install two or more plastic liners, and specifies the exact nature of the plastic to be used and the width to be used. That is a specification standard.

A design standard is one that specifies the use of a model technology that meets a legislatively articulated requirement, but design standards also permit individuals the freedom to achieve the same outcome by any other means. As noted, air and water pollution goals are usually stated in terms of a best available technology. The Environmental Protection Agency (EPA), for example, chooses a pollution limitation based on the amount of abatement that can be achieved by the current best available technology. A regulated entity, however, may use any abatement method as long as it will reduce pollution to the level of the model best available technology.

A performance standard is stated in terms of some regulatory goal. It does not specify the method that must be used to achieve that goal. For example, the Occupational Safety and Health Administration (OSHA) has set a limit on the amount of accumulated grain dust in grain elevators to reduce the risk of explosion. An elevator may choose any method it wishes to reduce dust to the specified level, as long as it meets that regulatory goal.

PROPOSED ALTERNATIVES TO COMMAND-AND-CONTROL

Some of the suggested alternatives are based on market incentives. Regulations can be written to take advantage of market-based or financial incentives to direct behavior toward a regulatory goal. This approach includes the following options:

1. *Taxes or charges.* Under this strategy, the regulator imposes a tax or a charge on the behavior to be regulated. For example, the government might tax each pound of a particular pollutant at a flat or even an escalating rate. Other examples include bottle deposits, increased gasoline taxes, or even higher taxes on old cars that pollute more.

2. *Liability provisions.* This approach requires a regulated entity or person to pay damages attributed to the harm that the entity or person has caused. Although liability regimes have notorious problems, modified approaches, such as no-fault compensation, might be used. For example, the focus of malpractice litigation might be shifted from individual physicians to the health organizations under whose auspices they practice.

3. *Information reporting.* This approach requires regulated entities to report certain kinds of information to the public, which in turn can create political and legal pressure via liability provisions to reduce risks. OSHA, for example, requires employers to distribute a Material Safety Data Sheet concerning each chemical or toxic substance to which a worker is exposed. Under the Clean Water Act, companies must file monthly Discharge Monitoring Reports that are public, and indicate the extent to which that firm is polluting.

4. *Subsidies, grants, and tax breaks.* These provide various forms of financial assistance from the government.

5. *Technical assistance.* These programs provide government advice and technical help to induce targeted entities to prevent or reduce pollution.

The final set of reforms that appear in the literature deal with voluntary approaches, of which two should be mentioned here:

1. *So-called "challenge regulations."* Under this approach the government identifies a goal and gives targeted entities time to select and implement effective means of achieving that goal. In back of this challenge lies the implicit threat that, "If you do not do something, we will regulate." For example, in the early 1980s OSHA adopted several enforcement programs that promised reduced inspections for voluntarily achieving below-average workplace injury rates. In the late 1980s, as another example, EPA established the 35-50 Program, in which companies that emitted 17 targeted toxic chemicals were challenged to reduce their emissions by 50 percent by 1995.

2. *"Consensus standards."* This approach has an agency using industry-generated standards as the basis for regulation. For example, the regulation of many toxic substances under OSHA's jurisdiction is based on permissible exposure limitations recommended by the American Council of Governmental Industrial Hygienists.

Serious consideration should be given to these regulatory alternatives. Yet, at the same time, it can be argued that the status quo has not performed as badly as many of its critics contend. Moreover, the alternatives that reformers have proposed are hardly perfect themselves. Critics have succeeded in exposing the maladies of current approaches to regulation for all to see, and from a distance, their alternative approaches look better by comparison. A closer look at the alternatives, however, reveals that they also pose implementation problems.

The correct public policy question, therefore, remains "Which method of regulation produces the fewest problems in reaching the intended regulatory goal?" As Neal Komisar has aptly concluded, "In a society of millions of persons with ever-changing technology, selecting the best means of preventing injury means carefully considering and comparing highly imperfect alternatives."

Specific Techniques

David Pritzker

The Administrative Conference of the United States (ACUS) is a federal agency, although a tiny one. It has been in existence for more than 25 years, for the purpose of studying administrative procedures and for advising the U.S. Congress, federal agencies, and the President on improving those procedures.[1]

ACUS STUDY AND RECOMMENDATIONS

ACUS has been studying various problems of administrative procedure. Some of these are quite narrowly focused and some are very broad based. In the late 1970s ACUS studied governmental use of voluntary consensus standards. That investigation disclosed a substantial private-sector engine that had been generating standards for many decades. There was a time, for example, when fire companies' hoses might not hook up to different sources of water because they were not all the same size.

A standards development industry thus arose. Through the 20th Century the industry has grown to encompass a variety of standards such as technical, safety, health, library, data and handling standards, among others. Many of these came into being by bringing together a committee of experts (or of purported experts), sometimes with a balance of manufacturers or producers and those who were buyers or users.

This is the model that ACUS had in mind in the early 1980s when it promulgated its recommendations to Congress and federal agencies on regulatory negotiation (sometimes called negotiated rule-making or "reg-neg"). The model was, in appropriate circumstances, to bring together a committee of representatives who could speak not necessarily by authority of particular

---

[1]Subsequent to this presentation Congress provided no FY96 funding for ACUS, which halted all operations 30 September 1995. David Pritzker is now with the Regulatory Information Service Center, and continues to provide information on regulatory alternatives for federal agencies.

interest groups but who could represent the points of view of the different interests affected.

THE ADMINISTRATIVE PROCEDURE ACT

Understanding of how this model evolved requires knowledge of some historical facts. In the 1940s Congress passed the Administrative Procedure Act, a recognition that Congress and the courts could not do everything that the people wanted the federal government to do. Numerous agencies were in existence by then, and many more were established in the succeeding decades, particularly in the areas of health, safety, and the environment. The Act passed by Congress in the 1940s established the ground rules for how these agencies were to work.

Agencies have a quasijudicial function (so-called adjudication), and they have a quasilegislative function (so-called rule-making). The Administrative Procedure Act requires the agencies, when they are considering the adoption of a rule, to let the public know through an announcement in the *Federal Register* that the agency has identified the problem, to give some indication (which might be quite brief or it might be quite extensive and detailed) as to what the agency is thinking about doing about the problem, and then to give the public an opportunity to submit its comments, generally in writing. This is called a Notice of Proposed Rule-making.

The Act does not specify how much time the agency must give the public to respond. In some instances, either through other legislation or through subsequent court decisions, agencies were required to give the public an opportunity for an oral hearing, particularly if the public asked for it. Essentially all the agency must do, however, is to say what it has in mind, give the public an opportunity to respond, and then publish a notice of a final rule-making containing the text of the rule and an explanation of how it responded to the comments that had been received.

Often, that is not the end of it, because those who do not like the regulations can go to the federal courthouse and try to do something about it. This is largely what has been tying the process up.

THE ALTERNATIVE: NEGOTIATION

To address this problem ACUS had in mind creating, in some instances, a committee that could try to "negotiate" a rule. This is not simply a process of turning regulation over to a committee that would largely comprise private citizens, and thus an abdication of agency responsibility. It is a procedure that gives people with different viewpoints about the problem—and about what the solutions might be—an opportunity to talk with each other in a public session in which the agency participates. The group would have incentives to come to agreement—primarily, that if they did not agree, the agency would make the decision by itself.

The objective was to offer to people of goodwill an opportunity to recognize the legitimate needs of the others represented and to see if through a negotiating process, including with the agency, a consensual resolution in the public interest could be achieved.

RECENT DEVELOPMENTS AND THE FEDERAL ADVISORY COMMITTEE ACT (FACA)

A number of agencies have tried the regulatory negotiation process, with some success. In 1990, to encourage its further use and to answer some of the legal questions that had been raised, Congress passed the Negotiated Rule-Making Act of 1990. Increasing numbers of agencies have been trying it ever since. The National Performance Review under the Clinton Administration has called for greater use of this technique. Figure 1 puts the negotiation process in a broader context of ways to build consensus.

Several consultation and consensus building approaches is available to the regulatory agencies, a number of which are in use by the Food and Drug Administration (FDA). Figure 1 notes the significance of the Federal Advisory Committee Act (FACA). FACA was passed about 20 years ago for the purpose of regulating the establishment and behavior of advisory committees created by statute or by the federal agencies to get advice. The problem that FACA was trying to solve was a proliferation of uncontrolled advisory committees that might be acting behind closed doors. Essentially, FACA now guarantees that the proceedings of advisory committees are open to the public, and it regulates other aspects of a committee's work. A committee that is subject to FACA cannot operate confidentially, for example, and must observe certain requisites of form and process. For example, with certain exceptions for matters of national security, a FACA committee must hold open meetings.

What that means is that if a committee is dealing with the public's business, there may be some limitations on the ability of the members of the committee to meet privately outside of the publicly announced schedule. That has been a problem that we have had to deal with in the negotiated rule-making context, since these negotiating groups are usually FACA committees. When Congress considered the Negotiated Rule-Making Act, it was urged to make modifications to FACA to facilitate the ability of the committee members to negotiate, but Congress was not enthusiastic about doing so.

	ONE-TIME MEETING				SERIES OF MEETINGS		
		Information Exchange			Consensus-Oriented Dialogue and Negotiation		
Public Hearings	Public Meetings	Single-Interest Consultations	Workshops and Forums	Roundtables and Informal Policy Dialogues	FACA Policy Dialogue	Regulatory Negotiation
		Standard APA Notice and Comment Procedure with Ad-Hoc, One-on-One Consultation				
Foundation					Foundation	
Relatively Formal		Relatively Informal			Relatively Formal	

FIGURE 1 Spectrum of consultation and consensus-building approaches available to federal agencies. Note: the vertical shaded bar is the "FACA line."

The objective of regulatory negotiation is usually to develop the actual text of the rule rather than only general principles or policies to guide the agency in its own drafting of a rule. The process is thus at the FACA-governed end of the scale.

Examples of techniques that are subject to the act are illustrated to the right of the shaded vertical line. In some cases roundtables or informal policy dialogues may in time become preferred sources of advice for the agency, and therefore fall under FACA.

Outside of FACA coverage are the relatively informal types of procedures, which can be forums, workshops, or consultations with single interests or more formal but one-time consultations, which can be either announced public meetings or public hearings that may have the formalities and additional procedure of cross-examination or other protection and that can perhaps be opportunities to respond to what the speakers have said at the hearings. Agencies can use a variety of techniques to develop consensus.

AUDITED SELF-REGULATION

ACUS is currently conducting a two part study of alternatives to direct regulation by federal agencies. The first half of the study led to a recommendation, adopted in June 1994, under the heading "use of audited self-regulation." In some industries and for some sectors of the economy it has proved to be workable and effective for an agency, under congressional authorization, to delegate to private, self-regulatory organizations the ability to implement and enforce laws or regulations, with the agency retaining the power of independent action and review. Among the best-known examples of this audited self-regulation are the stock and commodity exchanges. They in turn are monitored and audited by the Securities and Exchange Commission and the Commodity Futures Trading Commission.

These regulatory schemes have generally been fairly successful. They have also been applied in a number of other settings, including standards of medical care under government insurance programs, agricultural marketing agreements, certification of medical testing laboratories, and others. ACUS's work was directed at identifying the procedures that would ensure that they would work well, that is, both effectively and fairly. Effectiveness seemed to require finding a private group, the self-regulatory organization, with both the ability and the incentive to carry out the regulatory program. The agency also had to have the ability and the incentives to oversee the process and make it work. This included the need for substantive expertise on both sides. On the part of the agency, this includes knowledge of organizational behavior as well as the statutory authority to engage in this form of delegation.

As for fairness, the self-regulatory organization had to have sufficient procedural protection to constrain it to behave essentially as the agency would with respect to the regulated community and the public. Control would initially lie with the private organization, with periodic monitoring and right of appeal to the agency in case of improper behavior.

ACUS is now examining a further step: What safeguards are needed when there is no such self-regulatory private organization? There are different terms for this—self-implementation and sometimes self-enforcement—although the essence is the government's reliance on agents or employees of the regulated entities themselves to interpret and enforce the applicable laws and regulations, with the agency again being limited to monitoring the effort.

The private entities must have sufficient incentives to want to comply with the rules. Current research involves looking at what these incentives might be. For example, a regulated entity that has undergone a markedly successful inspection might be exempted from inspection again for a longer period of time instead of annually or biannually. Other self-regulatory schemes are built around reporting requirements. If the regulated firm reports its own violation, the potential penalties would be mitigated. The incentive systems are important ingredients in many such regulatory schemes.

Negotiated Rule-Making

Philip Harter

When considering alternative regulatory approaches it is important to ask not only whether it will work but also whether it is politically acceptable. The structure of negotiated rule-making (Reg-Neg) is a response to both sets of considerations.

"REG-NEG"—DOES IT WORK?

What is the experience with negotiated rule-making? Does this idea of empaneling a group of affected people and the agency to negotiate a rule actually work? The answer is yes, in numerous instances, of which several examples may be instructive.

Recently, the reformulation of gasoline to reduce toxic emissions was a negotiated rule. The Clean Air Act required a dramatic reduction. The Environmental Protection Agency (EPA), however, realized that, politically, the agency could not get a rule out through traditional rule-making. Thus, it empaneled representatives from the refiners, the auto industry, clean air advocacy groups, environmental groups, and the states. Over a 4-month period, the group did indeed develop the formula for reformulated gasoline.

To focus on how the process works, consider another example, the Federal Aviation Administration's (FAA's) rule involving pilot flight duty status time. FAA regulates how long pilots can fly, how long they must rest, how many hours a month they can fly, and the like. The original duty time rule, issued in 1947, was found in two paragraphs in the *Code of Federal Regulations*. In 1947 the pilots were former B-25 pilots fresh from World War II. They were 25 years old. They flew DC-3s nonstop all the way from New York to Philadelphia.

Over the years, things changed: DC-3s became 747s, the 25-year-olds became 65-year-olds, and the route became nonstop to Tokyo. The situation became very different, with many different demands placed on the pilot. FAA attempted to effect the necessary changes, but every time that it promulgated a proposal, if it favored the pilots the airlines had the wherewithal to block it. If it favored the airlines, pilots had the power to block it. FAA was stopped dead in its tracks. Unable to issue a new rule, FAA began to issue interpretive bulletins. Over time, what had been a two-paragraph rule became a set of interpretations of more than 1,000 pages.

FAA, having heard about negotiated rule-making but dubious about the probability of success, created a negotiating committee and set to work. Its doubts were based on the failures of the industry and agency to come to terms in the past; the issue seemed too controversial. Then, an odd thing happened in that committee. They agreed. They were able to talk about the real practical needs in the cockpit and the needs of the pilot—topics that had not been open to discussion before. For example, the pilots coming in from Paris land at Kennedy Airport, but there is no good place to stay at Kennedy Airport. They have to go into the city, adding another half hour to flight duty time. Now, every time that you get in an airplane you are trusting your life to a negotiated rule.

Another example is the ongoing negotiation of rules for the construction of steel buildings. The Occupational Safety and Health Administration (OSHA) looked at the various statistics, from which it was clear that the construction of steel buildings was probably the most hazardous occupation outside of mining. The agency's first response was that everybody who is exposed to a fall of more than 6 feet should be tied off. Interestingly, both industry and the union showed that it would be hazardous to tie off the first people who tie the structure together. They really ought to have freedom up to 30 feet.

One of the people on the committee said, "It is really pretty interesting that those guys don't fall. All the accidents are either above 30 feet, where people are already violating the existing rule, or below 10 feet, which is where the safety precautions really kick in, or doing something else." Getting the people together at the table to talk about how to build a building, what the needs are, and where the real risk is changed the perspective of the regulatory agency fundamentally—something that can occur only through this kind of direct dialogue.

THE PUBLIC AT THE NEGOTIATION TABLE

The beginning of negotiated rule-making is a sophisticated analysis of the kinds of interests at stake (who is substantially affected by the rule) and then the selection of representatives of those interests. Creativity sometimes is needed to identify members of the general public. For example, in the reformulated gasoline rule, who could represent everybody who drives? No one is going to spend 6 months of their life negotiating a rule to save $200 a year; yet, someone who can aggregate those interests and represent the common approach must be found.

The answer in this case turned out to be farmers. Gasoline is a major cost for their business, they are certainly well organized, and they are certainly aggressive in protecting that interest. Therefore, farmers were at the table to represent people interested in gasoline costs. The regulatory agency was also represented at the table, participating in the give and take of it and working toward a consensus on the recommended rule.

CONSENSUS

The goal of the process is consensus. For the purposes of a negotiated rule, "consensus" means that each interest represented at the table concurs—basically, unanimity. Each interest that participates has a veto.

Although critics of the process have expressed doubts about the workability of this process, it in fact has two major beneficial effects. First, if each interest has a veto, it is safe to come to the table. Recall the flight duty rule: each side had enough power to make sure that the agency could not issue rule that it did not like. Neither side however, had enough power to force it to issue a rule that it did like. A veto allows protection in the same way.

The second effect is that the group develops to some degree a "lifeboat mentality." Each party may feel about the other, "I do not like you very much and I hope I never see you again after we reach the island, but you know, we are not going to reach the island unless we row together." It converts the committee from a group of disparate interests into one with a common problem: How are we going to write a rule that reconciles all of these divergent interests within the statutory prescription?

It also has the effect of forcing people to look at the rule as a whole, as opposed to its individual parts. Negotiating rules is akin to buying a house. You may feel that a particular house is a great house but it has a bad yard, or it is a great house but you do not like the kitchen, or it is a great house but it needs another bathroom, or it is a great house but. . . . Unless one is exquisitely unimaginative, there is always something wrong with a house.

Then there comes a time when some house must be bought. Resource constraints are realities. The perfect house is not available. For every house, there are going to be parts you do not like. The same goes for a rule. All of this comes with the definition of consensus.

DECISION-MAKING DYNAMICS

In traditional technical data-based rule-making, people fight over the facts. Each interest argues that the facts prove that they are right. Why do they do that? They do it because they do not have control of the decision. They do it to constrain the discretion of the decision-maker. The facts are pushed well beyond what the science and technology can bear, and the parties are on the fringe of what is unknowable. In negotiating a rule the question is, how much information does a group of knowledgeable people really need to make a responsible decision?

It is usually possible to get rid of the 10 or 20 percent fringe. For example, the OSHA limit on occupational exposure to benzene had been kicked around for 9 years. OSHA issued the benzene standard, it went to the U.S. Supreme Court, and the Supreme Court reversed it and sent it back. OSHA then tried to negotiate it.

When the people got together they talked about that history. It had been going on for about 9 years, but that group of people, all the prominent people for all the interests, had been in the same room together only once before—and that was when they heard the oral arguments in the Supreme Court, where they certainly did not talk to each other. In the negotiating process, everyone was together, talking to each other for the first time.

As to the central issue of exposure limits, it was very clear that a dose-response curve for benzene would never be resolved. It is still being fought out in the technical journals. One of the parties then said, "We are never going to agree on the facts. The question is, what are we going to do about it? What is a responsible regulatory approach to it?" That turnaround is critical. It allows the parties to grapple with the real concerns of the driving policy on the basis of what can be agreed upon.

BENEFITS OF COLLABORATION

Negotiated rules tap very practical insight. Very practical people from the shop floor may be involved, and not just those from an agency who are necessarily distant from the action, working with derivative knowledge. The participants are people who are actually doing the work. They are then probed by others who are concerned about it.

Again, the reformulated gasoline process offers an example. The Clean Air Act prescribed one number for the evaporation limits. The petroleum industry, however, kept advocating for a very high number, that is, for highly volatile gasoline. Yet, it became clear that they could manufacture gasoline that was much less volatile. Through the probing and discussion among the group, it emerged that what the oil companies were really concerned about was that they could not achieve an effective limit on a gallon-for-gallon basis. Feed stocks differ, there are different kinds of equipment in the refinery, and some old material remains in the pipelines. However, they certainly could make it on the average. Hence the solution: the rule provides a very low number and very reduced volatility *on average*.

Here was a creative approach that could not have been done before. It could not have been done through notice and comment, and it probably could not have been done in legislation because it took a long time to figure out what the real problem was and how to fix it.

POLITICAL CONSENSUS

There is a further benefit to the negotiated rule-making process. Representatives of the parties sit at the table, haggling it out, and at the end they find an agreement. Although they are building the technical rule, they are also building a political consensus. That means that people are not going to endrun the rule to the Congress or challenge it in the courts.

Of the 20 or 30 negotiated rules—and they tend to be the most controversial ones—there has so far been only one challenge to a rule in which an agreement was reached, and that is in a bizarre setting. Again, it was the reformulated gasoline rule. After the rule had been negotiated, one of the producers of ethanol persuaded President Bush to overturn EPA, which he did in the final throes of an election. There are some people who have used this example as a criticism of the process, but in fact it is not. What happened in fact was that the committee came back together and persuaded the new President to overturn the old President, with one change. The parties to the original negotiation are now suing EPA to put the rule back to the way it was originally. In effect, the process had built the political consensus.

REG-NEG OUTCOMES

The result of the negotiation process is anything but a least-common-denominator approach. Interestingly, a negotiated rule is usually significantly more stringent than the one that the agency would have issued on its own, and yet, it is cheaper to implement.

How can that be? The result is practical. The agency knows where the shoals are and what to avoid. Everyone learns what is wasteful. The averaging in the reformulated gasoline rule would have never been done if it were a rule made by the agency. If EPA had issued that rule on its own, the Reid vapor pressure of reformulated gasoline would very likely have been somewhere halfway between what it is now and what was originally proposed, without any averaging. The air would have lost, and so would the refiners.

GETTING REG-NEG STARTED

What do we look for when we consider a Reg-Neg? Talk to the agency first, to get its description of the issues and the people who would be affected. Then talk to the people on that list. Ask everyone the same thing: what are the issues and who is affected? Frequently, the views of the private sector are very different from the agency's. Part of looking at the prospects of negotiated rule-making is issue definition.

For the process to work well there should be a limited number of interests that will be significantly affected, somewhere between 15 and 20. On the one hand that seems very small for a rule of major consequence. The burden, however, is usually carried by about that number of organizations. Caucuses will coalesce; it is not as small as it looks. On the other hand, 20 to 25 people can seem like a lot. It turns out that only five people talk anyhow, so it does boil down to a smaller number, but that larger number is still needed for representation.

The second thing to do is to identify appropriate individuals to represent those interests and to make sure that each issue, each major point, is discussed.

CHOOSING THE PROBLEM

The process works fairly well, although it does not work in all instances. There are conditions for likely success, and some degree of analysis is necessary to determine if the *issues* are of the sort for which a negotiated rule would be appropriate. This is the next question. Are the issues known, mature, and ripe for discussion? Nobody, let alone a committee, debates things in the abstract. Solving a problem that is not here yet is not a compelling circumstance. What this means is that the issue should be on the political agenda. The train is moving, something is going to happen. The decision-making process is beginning, and the outcome is on the horizon. One of the reasons for negotiating is to control that outcome.

OTHER REQUISITES

For the process to succeed, no party to it should have to compromise a fundamental value. This does not mean an important value; it means a value that is more like an article of faith. For example, no one could negotiate an end to the abortion issue right now or negotiate which of several religions is better.

Another criterion is that the issue should involve diverse aspects or elements. The essence of a negotiation is trading off one issue against another. For example, in the reformulated gasoline rule-making the petroleum companies agreed to a very stringent rule in return for an averaging process.

The next question is whether the outcome is really in doubt, whether there is a countervailing power. People do not negotiate if they can achieve their goals themselves. They come together in committees to control the outcome and to make sure that what they are concerned about is discussed. The pilots could not get what they wanted out of FAA. Neither could the airlines, nor could FAA. Everybody had a different kind of access. Some might have access to the White House, some have access to the Congress, and some have access to the *Washington Post*. It makes sense to come together to negotiate a truce in this war of attrition. If all of these conditions are met, the parties will likely view it to be in their interest to negotiate.

Last, and critically important, is the fact that the agency must be willing to rely on the process and to participate in it. Some agencies have been exquisitely creative in sabotaging things they do not like. As to whether this is an impermissible delegation of governmental authority to private individuals, the answer is "no." By the definition of consensus, everybody must agree—including the agency. As one senior agency official has said, "I am the one authorized by law to make the decision, but it does not invalidate my decision simply because everybody else agreed with me."

If the agency does not participate, the group will talk and talk until somebody gets tired and walks out, because the committee will not reach agreement. It is essential for the agency to be there.

CONSTITUENCY PRESSURES

As to the possibility that public pressure on the Congress is operating on the issues in question, the experience has been that once a committee is formed to address an issue, Congress usually does not intervene. If all of the constituents are sitting at the table saying that this is the forum in which to work it out, Congress tends to stay out of the loop. In several instances in which Congress was actively involved, the parties said, "We are finally solving the problem legitimately here and we will keep you posted." Several of the congressional representatives came to the first couple of meetings, and being confident that the issues were being addressed legitimately, they went away.

ACCOUNTABILITY

Before the agency engages in a negotiated rule, it publishes a notice in the *Federal Register* that it is about to engage in the process, usually with a list of the interests that would participate in it. That notice serves as an invitation to others to request participation. A few additional interests will often show up in this way, so save a few seats.

That initial public notice has two purposes. One is to make sure that anybody who is interested has an opportunity to participate. It also ensures that nobody can subsequently complain that they were not invited or that they could not participate. That is enormously important politically.

A critical part of the process is that all of the meetings be open to the public. Sometimes, if it is an area of considerable interest, there can be a lot of people, but the representatives get used to it after awhile and continue to talk candidly. This public openness makes an important contribution to accountability. People can see what is happening; people in the audience can present issues to be considered.

REG-NEG PROCESS

The following outline of the steps in a negotiated rule-making process was provided by David Pritzker:

1. Evaluation
   - Identify issues and deadlines.
   - Identify interested parties.
   - Compare with selection criteria.
   - Confirm management interest.
   - Select convener.

2. Convening, Phase I
   - Identify additional parties.
   - Discuss the negotiated rule-making process with parties.
   - Discuss issues with parties.
   - Determine willingness of parties to negotiate.
   - Report to agency.
   - Obtain agency management commitment.
   - Preliminary selection of 15 to 20 participants.

3. Convening, Phase II
   - Obtain parties' commitments to negotiate.
   - Publish Notice of Intent to Negotiate in *Federal Register*.

- Process Federal Advisory Committee Act (FACA) charter.
- Select a facilitator or mediator.
- Respond to public comments on the Notice.
- Adjust committee membership if necessary.
- Arrange organizational meeting.
- Arrange committee orientation and training.

4. Negotiations
   - Establish ground rules and protocols.
   - Define consensus.
   - Set meeting schedule.
   - Publish notices of meetings.
   - Review available information and issues.
   - Review draft rule or proposals.
   - Establish work groups or subcommittees.
   - Negotiate text or outline of proposed rule.

5. Rule-Making
   - Negotiations concluded.
   - If consensus is reached on language of rule:
     — Agency circulates draft for internal and external review.
     — Agency publishes consensus on draft rule.
   - If consensus is reached only on issues or outline:
     — Agency drafts proposed rule.
     — Agency circulates draft for internal and external review.
     — Agency publishes Notice of Proposed Rule-Making (NPRM).
   - If consensus is not reached:
     — Agency proceeds with rule-making with discussions as guide.
     — Agency drafts and publishes NPRM.
   - Draft rule is subject to public comment.
   - Committee is notified of public comments.
   - Agency revises rule if necessary.
   - Agency publishes final rule.

QUESTIONS ABOUT REG-NEG

Question: Who decides whether an issue deserves a guideline, a recommendation, or a regulation: the industry, the agency, or the public? Who is it that does the negotiating? Who represents the industry and the other interests? How is the venue established, and the shape of the table determined? What is the work product of the negotiation? How does an agreement get established? Does the requirement of unanimity reduce the likelihood of success?

David Pritzker: As to who decides who is going to be there, in a technical sense, under the provisions of the statutes, the agency ultimately decides. As a practical matter, however, the way that it has actually worked is that the agency or someone on behalf of the agency talks to the interested parties, and through these consultations, specific suggestions emerge as to who might best be representative of the different points of view. It has usually worked better if, in such consultations, the agency decides what organizations or what interest groups should be represented and then leaves it to the groups or the organization to determine exactly who will come to the table.

As to how appropriate issues are determined, like so many other things, it depends. To the extent that the agency knows the issues that it wants the group to address, the agency can say what it has in mind. If they have some general ideas but are not sure which ones the group could best work at, it can ask for their opinion, either before the process gets started or once the committee has been convened. Always bear in mind that this process is a *flexible* tool.

In part the choice of issues may depend on how well formed the agency's ideas are. If they are less well formed and they either want—or for political or other reasons are being pressed to have—that question decided by the other nonagency participants, that is okay, too. The process is broad enough to allow for the politics of the situation. Ideally, the entire group, including the agency, should come to a consensus on which issues will be negotiated.

As Phil Harter just mentioned, one of the criteria for Reg-Neg success is the outcome is genuinely in doubt. The issues are known and ripe for a decision. Those are questions for the agency and the other interested participants to explore. The process is broad enough to deal with various combinations. The notion of the convening process is that of an exploration that the agency starts to determine what is out there. Given all of these factors, the ultimate decision on whether to use reg-neg is simply whether it makes sense to bring together a committee to try to work out the issues. There is no black-and-white rule as to who decides what. Once the committee is together, the committee must be able to arrive at some consensus about its agenda and the nature of the consensus they are seeking on the rule itself. The flexibility should be fully stressed, for some of the regulatory agencies believe that the process has much less flexibility than is the case. In fact, an agency can mold this to its needs and its particular circumstances.

"Unanimity" and "veto" also need to be properly understood. Everyone at the table does have a theoretical veto. What that means in practice, however, can be different. First, the group could agree to proceed without the requirement of unanimity. Assume that unanimity is required and that the group has debated for many months but all members cannot agree. Suppose the count is 24 to 1. Does the group have consensus? No. What is the agency going to do?

INNOVATIONS AND ALTERNATIVES

That depends on what the committee is willing to have the agency do and what the agency decides to do in the absence of consensus.

If the basis for the negotiations is "if you don't have unanimous agreement you have nothing," then there is no consensus. What the agency does have, however, is the experience and the record of the negotiations. It knows what the issues are, it knows the feelings of the group as a whole, and it knows the feelings of the individual representatives of the constituencies. The agency is now free to do what it will, but in general, the agencies that have found themselves in those circumstances have come forth with rules based on the majority view. On a couple of occasions they have been sued, but for the most part the courts readily upheld the agency's rule. The standard traditionally used in court is whether the agency acted arbitrarily and capriciously. It is likely to be difficult to show that the agency was arbitrary when it has been through this negotiation process and has only one or two holdouts. The agency has the benefit, even if it does not have consensus, of having heard the debate. It has heard suggestions for solutions to the problems, and it has heard the responses. It knows what the real-world consequences are likely to be. That is what happens in practice.

Panel Discussion on Applications of Negotiated Rule-Making to Issues in Blood Banking

Kathryn C. Zoon: It has been helpful to have the opportunity to discuss these issues regarding FDA and its regulatory responsibilities. The mission of the Center for Biologics Evaluation and Research (CBER) is to protect and enhance the public health through the regulation of the products for which it is responsible, and to make those products available. Whatever regulatory course is taken and whatever changes may ultimately be made, that mission will not change.

With that preface, it is worth noting that the discussion of regulatory alternatives actually relates to a number of areas that CBER and other FDA components have discussed of late—new regulatory paradigms.

REGULATORY INITIATIVES AT FDA

I would like to share with you some of the initiatives currently being taken by CBER, and how they integrate with broader initiatives such as government streamlining/government reinvention, including the National Performance Review activities.

CBER has begun a strategic planning process. Some very important and fundamental issues continue to be in our minds. One is a reaffirmation of science-based decision making. If we lose sight of the science in regulation, the public health's interests are not well served.

We also need to examine how we are using our resources. With downsizing and refining how we do business, the expectations are not to do less in all cases. We need to be creative and still fulfill the mission, but to do it with less. That creates some challenges and controversies with respect to a number of areas.

We are also looking at partnerships. As we go into the next decade, the ability and the need to rely on partnerships—partnerships within the government, partnerships with industry, and partnerships with academia—in order to effect useful and important regulations to protect the public health, become very critical. We see this now in a number of our international harmonization efforts. We have been actively engaged in partnerships. Those partnerships will continue to exist and will be enhanced. We need to have outside input to understand what the agency is asking people to do, how we do that, and how in the end we can serve the public in terms of having a blood supply in which they feel confident.

We must think globally. We do not live in an isolationist community where decisions made outside our country do not affect us. We must become more involved in those decisions and become partners in making those decisions. They affect the area of blood regulation as well as the other areas that come under our regulatory purview. This is true for FDA as a whole; CBER is not unique from that point of view.

FDA IN THE FUTURE

In our strategic planning process, as we look to the year 2004, we see a more closely managed center, one in which our processes are defined and managed to set up level playing fields, internal and external. It is important for our own staff as well as people in the outside communities to be able to work and interact and have input into the agency. That is very important in public decision-making.

We see that this transcends not only our regulatory processes but also our research processes. Focusing and enhancing their contributions to our regulatory mission will continue to evolve. It is important to have public confidence. We cannot stop trying to regain public confidence if it is not where it should be. That is a job that for all of us—people in the blood banking industry, and people in the government. If we need to take steps to do that, then that is part of our job.

For us to do our business more effectively and more efficiently, we also see the need for information management systems. Again, in times of limited resources the ability to deal with the issues will require an interactive database in which information can be drawn not only from our own agency but also from other sources inside and outside the federal government. We need to be able to adapt and manage that, and to share that information where appropriate.

INITIATIVES AT CBER

A number of specific initiatives are going on at CBER. One involves the re-write of the general biologics regulations, as well as the blood regulations. This is an excellent opportunity to look at our processes and the flexibility of our regulatory structure. Some of our rules and regulations that may have served their purposes decades ago are now outdated and need more flexibility.

Science continues to move at a rapid pace in the area of biologics. To keep up with that pace, one needs to be able to make adaptations relatively quickly and to not be confined by changes in rule-making, which tend to be very cumbersome. Over the years we have tried to use workshops, "points to consider" documents, and memoranda in a more flexible fashion. There are ups and downs to all of these things. Alternatives are never perfect, and we keep looking for ways to improve the ability to get input, to communicate and have decision-making based on scientific data as well as other factors that affect a particular area under discussion.

In the next 5 to 10 years the focus on performance-based management will be our future. Under the National Performance Review, some of our initial negotiations with industry in developing the user fee program for new prescription drugs provide an example of not quite negotiated rule-making for the agency, but this is probably as close as we have come to collaborative discussion of what we thought would help improve processes as well as performance. It has had a lot of benefit to the public, the industry, and the agency.

WILLINGNESS TO EXPLORE PILOTS

FDA has not been reluctant to do pilot projects to examine new regulatory paradigms. That is still the case, although in fairness, while issues have been raised about FDA regulation, I do not perceive the process and the results of the process to be broken. Our processes have served the public health in this country, but that does not mean that we cannot look at new ways of doing business and making it better. At the end of the analysis, are we willing to look at and evaluate how we do our business? I believe the answer to that is "yes."

In order to have a good and effective pilot project there are several things we need to do. One is to define clearly what the pilot should address. Two, the pilot should have substantial public health impact. Three, it would need to be viewed as something that is useful.

It is important not only to develop the pilot project, but also to do an evaluation of the pilot. Has it been effective? Then one must determine whether or not those changes are doing what you anticipated they would do: Are they making it better? Are they making it worse? Have they made no change at all? Although one can experiment, as with any experiment one needs to evaluate the information critically and decide what has been learned and gained. That way one can then apply the process to other areas and other issues with the expectation that it will have a positive impact. What I would like to see is some discussion of areas and targets that might be pilot experiments that we can bring back to our organization and discuss candidly.

The discussion brought up here is certainly the beginning of a dialogue. I look forward to continuing the dialogue. The issues raised about negotiated rule-making are intriguing, and require additional thought and discussions with this group as well as within CBER. Further discussion will occur, within FDA and between FDA and other organizations. I welcome those discussions.

Jay Epstein: Kathryn Zoon has described the broad initiatives. I would like to embellish a few points, with some particulars in the area of blood regulation.

INITIATIVES IN BLOOD REGULATION

The regulation review process is ongoing to identify sections of the regulations that require updating. The ongoing debate is whether we should create additional standards for specific products under the regulations or move toward more flexible models of regulation such as those described during this Forum. In that discussion a lot is at stake for the future of regulation.

A set of initiatives is related to report reduction. This was started under the pharmaceutical drug user fee negotiation, but it is clearly on the agency's agenda to extend it to the area of blood regulation. The idea is to determine the minimum necessary change requiring reporting and determine what requires prior approval versus what can be implemented with a subsequent report to the agency. This is an area particularly relevant to the implementation of computerized systems, when the blood banks do not want to be at the agency's doorstep for every minor tinkering or fix.

There are other initiatives, for example increasing exemptions from lot release. That is an issue which, in the area of blood and blood products, will mainly focus on diagnostic tests. We find ourselves, however, repeatedly dealing with the question of shortages because of the impact of FDA control procedures, and a lot of that discussion tends to focus on lot release and how we should use lot release generally versus how we should control particular problems. This is an area that needs a sound debate.

The computerized product license application review is another fruitful area, not only because of the possibility of expediting review procedures through the use of information management technology but also because of the goal of reducing at least part of the applications procedure to automated checklists. We have an initiative related particularly to the source plasma application in that domain.

Another example of creativity in the area of streamlining has to do with the delegation of responsibility for inspections. The agency has been moving toward more reliance on the field offices to play a primary role in inspections other than the prelicense approval inspections. The idea is to create a more homogeneous vantage point for the field with respect to the entire agency in looking across the board at inspection-related issues and trying to concentrate expertise in an appropriate way.

Managed review under the Pharmaceutical Drug User Fee Act (PDUFA), has also had a tremendous impact on other areas of regulation. It has already had an impact on forming time frames and developing performance standards in the area of blood regulation, particularly affecting devices.

Within the strategic planning process a similar concept is an attempt to have management take control over research so that research can be coordinated in a fashion that would focus it more on the mission of FDA.

PARTICIPATORY DECISION-MAKING

An issue intriguing issue is the role of negotiation—or perhaps in a broader construct, a more public decision-making process. Without having had in mind the formal negotiated rule-making (Reg-Neg) construct, which is very exciting, we have been moving in that direction as a response to the forces that have been acting upon us. I would cite as examples the degree to which we have been seeking to perform our regulatory duties by improving guidance statements and educating industry.

Other examples would include the quality assurance guideline that was developed through a workshop process and a similar guidance document on the validation of computer systems in the blood bank. Perhaps a less well recognized example is the fact that we have been taking error and accident analysis, which are done in the agency, and going public with them as a form of industry assistance through memoranda. We did that in March 1991 and will do that again periodically. Another model is using workshops to develop license standards. We have done this now for irradiated red cells, and we have the intention to do it with leuko-filtered blood components.

Another change that has been made concerns the way that we are using the Blood Products Advisory Committee. We received a great deal of industry comment about opening up that committee process and trying to use it as a communications tool. For example, we have deliberately brought new products before the advisory committee for discussion before products are approved.

We have taken very seriously the charge that industry is in an impossible position when it learns of a deadline on the day that the memorandum is published and has pressure to implement a major change within 48 or 72 hours. Instead, we are trying to give industry the "heads up" that it needs by making known the state of progress toward approval of critical new products to the advisory committee.

Another change has to do with using the advisory committee to discuss decision making related to risk assessment and risk management. We have been doing this quite consistently in the last decade, since the start of the AIDS era, and have applied that model to dealing with many issues.

Another change has been the way that we are using liaison meetings with the industry. We now have regular liaison meetings with more groups. That is not seen by the agency as a wonderful thing, because it tends to result in a proliferation of the number of meetings, and, some discussion of the subject matter tends to be repetitive. That aside, however, we have a regular liaison on the Transfusion-Transmitted Diseases Committee, regular liaison meetings with American Association of Blood Banks, and liaison meetings together and separately with the Council of Community Blood Centers and the American Blood Resources Association. We are benefitting from those meetings, as opportunities for the agency to listen and get the word from the "shop floor."

PUBLIC MEETINGS

The Center for Biologics, Evaluation and Research (CBER) has also been using public meetings as part of the conventional process of notice and comment rule-making. That effort has been proactive, in that we are trying much harder to identify the concerned interests and bring them to the table. We still must work through the mechanism of an open public hearing, but we are endeavoring to get the word out so that all of the concerns are heard at these meetings and we try not to make it a haphazard process in which the right people must read the notice in the *Federal Register*.

Another change has been the effort to broaden the representation on the Blood Products Advisory Committee. In the wake of the discovery of the human immunodeficiency virus (HIV) in the 1980s, there was an accusation that the advisory committee was too dominated by blood bank concerns and was not sufficiently responsive to consumer concerns. We have addressed that by revising the charter to add to the number of members permitted on the committee and have appointed special government employees, individuals with interest in particular sides of the issue who can function as consultants or guests of the committee. That has been the method, by which we have tried to increase the level of representation of the hemophilia community.

NATIONAL PERFORMANCE REVIEW

Under the National Performance Review we are expected to come up with performance standards for all of our activities. We have opened that process up to the blood industry by requesting specifically that the industry form some cooperating forum and get back to the agency on its recommendations and expectations for the performance standards to which the agency will hold itself.

What we are talking about, for example, is the standard defining the length of a product licensing application (PLA) review or a 510k[2] review, the percentage of such reviews accomplished within the time frame based on the resource. It is the same model as PDUFA but without any added external resource beyond the federal tax dollar. We have extended that opportunity to industry and advocated it at some of the liaison meetings.

EXPERIMENTS IN REGULATION

So far I have been describing ways in which we are trying to make the present system work better. We could do a lot more but we have already performed some experiments. I want to note a few of them.

First, there is the manner in which we are regulating the banking of human tissue. We do that under the Communicable Disease Control Authority of the Public Health Services Act Part 361, not under the Product Approval Authority of Part 351. That is a bit of an experiment because it is an alternative to device regulation.

Second, there is the issue of the extent to which CBER will elect to review more of the in vitro diagnostic devices under premarket approval versus product licensing application. That is an experiment because it shifts the balance of the establishment review from the preapproval stage to the field.

Third, there is the question of how far we will pursue good practice (GMP) regulation of unlicensed products. We tend to see this as an alternative to product review when we do not have licensing standards. We are engaging in an experiment in which we are trying to find ways of approaching vendor software and approaching human stem cells as a product subject to GMP, but not yet subject to a license review. We still have the mind-set that these products will become licensable once we understand the standard, but it is an experiment to try to achieve standards of safety under the GMP approach without the license review.

The impact of federal legislation dealing with risk assessment and cost-benefit analysis is uncertain. We have not ventured very far into that domain

---

[2] This is referred to in section 510k of the 1976 amendments to the Food, Drug, and Cosmetic Act. The provision allows FDA to approve a product for marketing without pre-market review provided that product is "substantially equivalent" to a device that was marketed prior to the passage of the 1976 amendments.

does cover risk benefit assessment, which we commonly discuss in our advisory committee proceedings, but except in the domain of rule-making, FDA is not supposed to engage in the discussion of cost per se. I think that is an important problem, and I think that much good discussion will come out of the proposed legislation, although at this point there is no official FDA response to it.

THE FORCES OF CHANGE

We are living in a complex world. There are international forces relating to harmonization, and there is the changing tide of congressional oversight, which, whether it is of liberal or conservative persuasion, is still very deterministic toward the activities of the agency.

We have the agenda of downsizing. We have the agenda of accountability under performance review. We have the conflicting agendas of using fewer resources, while performing regulatory activities and ensuring safety more effectively. I do not know how we will accomplish that balancing act, but examples of experimentation exist at FDA.

FDA has permitted the use of voluntary standards. For example, the question of whether to formally regulate the human tissue industry has been debated for almost 20 years. In the interim voluntary standards were accepted as the basis for self-regulation, and it was only in the wake of certain incidents such as HIV transmission by transplanted organs and tissues that a more formal regulatory approach has been taken.

The agency has a history of flexibility. What remains to be examined is the exact issues that are ripe for either negotiated rule-making or an alternative mode of regulation. That is where the thoughtfulness and effort need to be applied. It is not fundamentally an issue of rigidity of the agency. It is more a question of trying to define what our expectations are and to determine the specific areas where it is reasonable to try these novel approaches.

THE ROLE OF THE RULE-MAKING PROCESS

Question from the Audience: Two questions were put to Jay Epstein concerning the fact that FDA has not often used the "*Code of Federal Regulations* CFR process"—the formal notice-and-comment procedure for rule-making under the Administrative Procedure Act, but has, rather, relied more on issuing guidelines and recommendations than on promulgating rules. Thus, the following questions were asked. First, given the structure of Reg-Neg, could adopting it have the ironic consequence of causing a shift away from the informal structure of rule-making and back to the formal structure? Second, given the parallel tracks in FDA's regulatory activities, including both CFR rule-making and the recommendations and "points to consider procedures" involving public comment through the Blood Products Advisory Committee, is there not still a need for some alternative process, one that involves more rather than less negotiation, with the end products being decisions that come out not necessarily as rules in the CFR?

Jay Epstein: CFR-type rule-making has not been and could never be abandoned. But the agency has learned just how hard it is to get rules out, and so there is a higher threshold for engaging in formal rule-making.

The question is, at how many levels can you change the system. Under the current legal structure, agencies must promulgate regulations as the basis for their authorities. They derive their authorities from their governing statutes and then promulgate regulations on the basis of authority and, in the case of FDA, their authority for enforcement. That must remain as the agency's fundamental legal framework. The issue that we have addressed is what is the necessary level of detail in regulations for us to regulate effectively. A lively debate on that question is occurring. One camp contends that we should be more specific with our regulations because that is the only way to resolve the ambiguities that crop up with enforcement. How do you rein in compliance? The answer is, by specifying things more precisely in the regulations, and eliminating the ambiguity. The other argument is that when there are regulations written in that they do not stand up against the test of time. They become outdated; they tend to be too particular; there are too many circumstances not captured in the regulations. What one really wants are general framework regulations that then permit the agency to periodically issue and update interpretations that are enforceable. There is a debate about that, too, about how enforceable interpretations are. I do not have the answer to these things, but I do not see abandoning regulations in *CFR* as an endpoint that we can reach. I do think, though, that trying to develop flexible ways to use more spare regulations is a realistic end point.

Toby Simon: Even in the current political climate, blood bankers have not been opposed to regulation by FDA. There is a general consensus that regulation is an important part of the profession and that it is essential in many ways. To deal with the public it is important for FDA to be there, reassuring the public about the safety of blood by virtue of its activities.

In addition to the new regulatory tools already discussed, another one worth mentioning is "error management," looked at from the point of view of both the transfusion service and the blood center. The Federal Aviation Administration (FAA) has used reporting of near misses anonymously to encourage full reporting, and the reports are processed under FAA guidance to make sure that everybody knows of and can benefit from them.

Negotiated rule-making itself might allow us to move more rapidly in areas that we have been dealing with from a regulatory point of view, particularly in terms of inspection and enforcement. Likewise, self-audit with FDA review is an interesting concept. Today, GMP audit results are ordinarily not shared, theoretically to stimulate a complete investigation. One might take the opposite point of view and share the audit, having FDA determine whether the audit has been adequate and thereby improving the efficiencies of its inspection.

If asked to define the characteristics of an appropriate regulatory process for the issues facing us, I would suggest that one characteristic would be involvement. That is, there would be a significant input from different parties who have a potential impact—government, the private sector, patients potentially affected, and specialists in related areas (for example, infectious disease specialists and neurologists). We would have some way to bring that group together to formulate a consensus, and to have the flexibility to keep measuring what we do, to come back and look at it, and to change it again.

COMMENTS AND QUESTIONS

Question from the Audience: As a practical matter, there is an increased risk of civil liability when FDA issues a recommendation and a blood bank does not abide by it. Thus, in effect, the blood industry complies as fully with recommendations as with regulations. From FDA's point of view, do recommendations and guidelines have a potency or effect different from those of regulations themselves?

Jay Epstein: Because FDA does not make recommendations that are not within its authorities under the regulations or, in some fairly rare cases, direct interpretations of statutes, the agency would regard recommendations as enforceable to the degree that they are grounded in a regulation or statute. There are occasional challenges in court, and FDA does not always win.

Thomas Zuck: One difficulty with the present system, which a negotiated rule-making process might help to alleviate, is illustrated by the question of stem cells. The agency indicated that it was going to regulate stem cells and somatic cell lines. But then, whether it is by regulation or by guideline, there is a long period during which we do not know whether to file an investigational new drug (IND) application, whether to ship in interstate commerce, or whatever else we are supposed to do. In that kind of situation we have to wait

INNOVATIONS AND ALTERNATIVES 83

until somebody is cited for a violation or is brought to court. That is not a very good way to make rules. These alternatives offer a way to get on with it, to convene a process to decide.

Unidentified Participant: The present process is one in which FDA receives input and issues a decision. These negotiation alternatives allow all of us, and others who have an interest in the rule, to sit at the table together, communicate, and hammer out those guidelines and "points to consider."

James MacPherson: The present system is not serving us well, and we do not believe that it is serving the public well. Most of the current initiatives, about which I agree there has been progress, have largely been internal. It has so far been FDA creating policy entirely internally and then seeking comment. We should now be talking about a true partnership, not a partnership between FDA and the field office or between CBER and the field office, but a true partnership with all of the parties involved and in which there is no risk to anyone. The only risk is that we may fail again.

Pinya Cohen: Negotiated alternatives seem difficult but challenging and exciting; they could add substantial value to the regulatory process, particularly given the need for depoliticization. Politics and ideology have little to do with safety, yet the Commissioner's office has a need to respond to the U.S. Congress. There is really no need for a body like that to be active other than to monitor in a general sense what is going on. We can take the reins fully in our own hands if we hold ourselves to some new standards.

William Sherwood: We have heard in these Forums several looming issues. We have heard of the deterioration or the erosion of the public trust in our industry. We have heard that the public has a far more dire expectation or understanding of the safety of our blood supply compared with what we think it is. And we have discussed the regulatory environment that we are in and have looked at it as perhaps a problem. That question—dealing with the regulatory environment—is, at least from inside the industry, one of the most important.

Is the problem rule-making? As I look at the rules that have been made, I do not have much quibble. Rule-making has been slow: slow in coming and slow in eliminating rules that are there. Maybe that is a problem that can be corrected.

Are the issues more that of how the rules are applied? How they are interpreted by the agency? How they are laid out? Is there an unevenness or a lack of consistency in the way in which these rules are looked at, and is our industry kept off balance? These are issues and problems on which we can focus. Maybe now we have some alternatives that we can work with the agency to develop.

Pinya Cohen: With all due respect to the inspections in the field, there is a growing sense that there is a lack of coordination or a question as to who reports to whom with regard to the inspectors in the field. In the application process, we have certainly had a dialogue with CBER. But once our applications are approved, one gets the impression that the inspectors in the field may feel free to challenge and reopen that dialogue. If these are the ground rules, we should know them in a clear way. We need to pull together and get back to a more centralized sense of where the science is coming from. A science-directed approach rather than a compliance-directed approach might be helpful.

Miriam Sparrow: We have heard today about countervailing power, and we have heard about rule-making and the legislative function of FDA. It is the enforcement function of FDA, however, that we also need to work with, specifically, the inspection process, which does have a role to play in improving blood safety. Part of where we should be headed, in terms of trying to work together, is to build not only an FDA that has credibility with the public at large and with the congressional constituency, but also an FDA that has the same credibility with the industry that is being regulated. That objective will help the industry itself to meet some of the concerns about public perception.

Henrik Bendixen: How have advances in blood safety come about? Have we done it all ourselves? It is fair to say that we have done a lot ourselves, through the introduction of new concepts, good research, the introduction of more technology, and the writing of guidelines, standards, and the like. All of this has contributed to increased safety in our field. At the same time, we have not been alone. The intervention of professional societies has been very important. Then, of course, there has been attention from the press and the voices of the consumer and special interest groups, and we cannot deny that even lawsuits may have moved us in the right direction.

The other participating change agents have been regulations, whether they are those of the federal government or the states. Advances in safety do not logically argue toward deregulation. Nonetheless, as we live in a modern industrial society, a most important thing is the word "predictability." You need to have rules of the game. You do not mind even tough rules of the game as long as you know what the rules are. If McDonald's stops selling hamburgers in the People's Republic of China it will be because they cannot predict from one day to the next who has to be persuaded or bribed. I have never minded regulation, even tough regulation, but it must be predictable.

Jay Epstein: I would like to say "message received" with respect to the issue of integrating the enforcement side into these discussions. I see that as an area that could be developed as some kind of model for a negotiated resolution. The points made about accountability are also quite perceptive. Ultimately we are a federal agency; we are accountable to our leaders, to the U.S. Department of Health and Human Services, and ultimately to the Congress, and that should never be forgotten. As an example, increased role of the field offices in decision-making and policy generation is a direct result of congressional oversight, which faulted the agency for not responding enough to the role of the field in that process.

We cannot have it both ways; the implication is that there is a need for a careful examination of the political environment and figuring out who the constituents are and how they interact. The system must be looked at as a whole, and the players must be recognized. We must not forget that the Congress as the voice of the people is the ultimate master of the agency.

General Discussion of Issues for Negotiated Rule-Making

Editor's Note: A portion of a later meeting of the Forum was set aside for discussion of the topics that could be considered as candidates for a pilot project in negotiated rule-making. David Pritzker offered a checklist of qualifications that a candidate issue should have, Jay Epstein suggested the problem of new tests, and Celso Bianco presented the particular case of Creutzfeldt-Jacob disease (CJD). Other members of the Forum proposed specific candidate issues, a list of which follows. Consistent with its charter, the Forum as a group took no position on recommending any particular issue or program.

CRITERIA FOR SELECTING ISSUES

David Pritzker: The following is an amalgam of several of the published checklists describing the features of problems for which Reg-Neg seems most promising:

1. Both parties must be dissatisfied with the current situation.
2. There must be a limited number of interests that are significantly affected.
3. The appropriate individuals who can represent those interests can be identified.
4. The issues must be known, mature, and ripe for discussion.
5. No party should be able to reach the result by themselves—that is, the outcome is genuinely in doubt and no interest should be able to dominate the proceedings.
6. No party can be required to compromise a fundamental value.
7. The problem must involve diverse issues, so there are things to trade off.
8. The agency must be willing to rely on the process and actively participate in it.
9. The parties see it as in their interest to use the process.
10. There should be a deadline for achieving a result.

CANDIDATES FOR REG-NEG

Jay Epstein: One issue that has been pressing and that may be appropriate is development of a framework for dealing with changes in the institution of tests. The effort is to come up with a set of principles that can be used to work through the problems that have faced blood safety. There has been a sense that we have dealt ad hoc or case by case with issues, not always to the benefit of the system as a whole, and that there is a need to focus on the decision-making process—not perhaps to fault or revise the process as a system but to put it on a better foundation. That has been seen as one of our pressing issues. The structure of the regulatory agency-industry relationship is certainly another, but that is a little bit more long term than an effort to develop guiding principles for risk decision making.

Celso Bianco: CJD is an interesting problem for these models. At the Blood Products Advisory Committee in December 1994, we presented a model by which certain decisions could be made. The idea was that each blood center would report those diseases to a central place, for example, to the Food and Drug Administration, which would file them and once a year convene a panel of experts, including patients and others, and ask the questions, "Would notification of recipients of these products be beneficial to them? Is there anything known that could help them?" That is one example of a small pilot project that could encompass not only CJD but other diseases that are ill-defined. There are diseases for which there are theoretical possibilities of transmission by transfusion but for which there is no documented evidence of actual transmission.

The following are additional "Reg-Neg" topics suggested by members of the Forum:

- *Progenitor cells.* The technology is moving very fast.
- *p24 antigen testing for HIV.* For detection of HIV during the "window period" after infection but prior to detectable antibody response.
- *Recommendations concerning "lookback."* The cost and benefits; how the information is and is not used, whether lookback actually serves the recipient population.
- *Stem cells and gene therapy regulations.*
- *Transplantation regulations.*
- *Test implementation decision process:* implementing new tests and eliminating old ones. It would be desirable to establish a decision-making process outside of the "heat of battle." Specification of steps, timing, and procedures is needed.

- *Prevention of Chagas disease transmission.* This is linked to the issue of implementing new tests.
- *Organizational alternatives to current U.S. blood banking system:* federation (e.g., Scotland) or national blood banking system.
- *Definition and role of "donor incentives".*
- *Donor deferral and reentry.*
- *How should the safety of the blood supply be monitored?*
- *Regulation of new classes of products such as hemoglobin solutions*: safety and efficacy; adequacy of substrate supply.
- *Approval of significant blood-processing techniques:* virus inactivation; blood filtration.
- *Recipient screening.* Is this a practical solution, or a logistical nightmare?
- *Establishment inspections.* Increase uniformity of the inspection process; develop internal audits.
- *Computer validation*: computer models and quality systems; integration into the inspection process.

IV

Congressional Oversight and Regulatory Initiatives

Editor's Note: In July 1995, as the Forum on Blood Safety and Blood Availability was preparing the agenda for its final meeting, the Institute of Medicine (IOM) report *HIV and the Blood Supply* was issued. That report was a retrospective discussion of the events of the early and middle 1980s concerning transfusion-associated human immunodeficiency virus (HIV) and AIDS, with a special focus on decision-making. The authors of that study offered a number of recommendations to the Department of Health and Human Services (DHHS), to the blood banking industry, and to the public. The Forum therefore invited Anne Marie Finley and Mary Pendergast to address the closing session of the September 1995 meeting, to describe the work of the Congress and of the DHHS with respect those recommendations. Their presentations continue the theme of regulatory effectiveness and regulatory reform.

Congressional Oversight of Blood Safety Issues

Anne Marie Finley

On behalf of Chairman Christopher Shays, I am pleased to have the opportunity to discuss with you the work of the Human Resources and Intergovernmental Relations Subcommittee. The subcommittee has oversight jurisdiction over the U.S. Department of Health and Human Services (DHHS) and its agencies, including the Food and Drug Administration (FDA), the Centers for Disease Control and Prevention (CDC), and the National Institutes of Health (NIH), for the House Government Reform and Oversight Committee. Our oversight responsibilities in the blood safety area are taken very seriously not only because of the loss of life in the HIV epidemic but also because of our oversight obligations with regard to government reform.

THE WORK OF THE SUBCOMMITTEE

In May of 1995 the subcommittee began a general oversight investigation into blood safety issues and FDA's management of the Blood Products Advisory Committee. This investigation resulted in a letter from Chairman Shays to FDA Commissioner David Kessler requesting that the agency not accept the June 23rd recommendation of the Blood Products Advisory Committee (BPAC) but, rather, that FDA license a short-incubation HIV monoclonal p24 antigen test for donor screening.

The Chairman's concerns included prevention by up to 40 individuals per year from exposure to antigen-positive, antibody-negative blood products; continued incentives for the development of further screening tools to close the window period during which HIV infected persons test negative on the current antibody based test; and a determination "that cost estimates should not outweigh scientific evidence of the effectiveness of antigen testing to save lives." The Chairman also objected to the agency's failure to approve or disapprove the product licensing applications (PLAs) for the short-duration antigen tests within the 180 days mandated by the Federal Food, Drug and Cosmetic Act.

PLAs were initially filed in 1990 and remain unapproved and pending at the agency. Furthermore, Chairman Shays asked Dr. Kessler to disband the Blood Products Advisory Committee immediately and to replace it with an advisory committee on the safety of the nation's blood supply. He felt that the critical mission of this advisory committee should be reflected in its title and that its mission should be clear.

Consistent with HR 1021, legislation introduced by Representative Porter Goss, Chairman Shays stated that at least one third of the membership of the new advisory committee should be individuals who have received blood products or who are representatives of consumer organizations with expertise in blood products.

The subcommittee was very pleased with FDA's August 10, 1995, announcement, including the recommendation that blood establishments should begin screening all blood and plasma donors with the antigen test kits within 3 months after FDA's approval of the initial test kit.

On October 12, the Subcommittee will conduct an oversight hearing on DHHS's management of the risk of infectious agents in the blood supply. This will be a culmination of not only the antigen investigation but continuing work that we will be doing in blood. We expect testimony from DHHS officials, U.S. Public Health Service agency representatives, consumers, clinicians, and individuals from the regulated industries to address prospective problems in the regulatory scheme for blood and blood products. We do not expect to relitigate the incidents of the early 1980s, but we do anticipate testimony on the DHHS's response to the IOM recommendations. (*Editor's Note*: The IOM recommendations referred to by Ann Marie Finley are not those of the present IOM Forum, but of the IOM report *HIV and the Blood Supply*.)

Additional issues that concern the subcommittee and that may come up at blood investigations and hearings include emerging infectious agents in the blood supply, the status of antigen test kit reviews, reconstitution of the Blood Products Advisory Committee, and hepatitis C virus transmission through blood and blood products. There is a strong possibility that the way in which we regulate blood and blood products will change not only at the agency and department level but possibly through congressional and public interest as well.

Chairman Shays and the subcommittee share the commitment of the regulatory agencies, consumers, and the regulated industries to the safety of the blood supply and welcome efforts to develop responses to the recommendations of IOM so that the blood supply remains as free from infectious agents as strong leadership and good science can ensure.

THE QUESTION OF COSTS

Question from the Audience: We have many health crises in this country and very limited resources to deal with them. When does cost become an issue?

Anne Marie Finley: Under the current statute FDA has no authority to consider and make regulatory decisions based on cost effectiveness. Their only criteria are safety and efficacy. We were concerned that the antigen testing issue at BPAC was, in fact, decided on some other basis. Whether that resulted from improper instruction with regard to what the criteria were or whether the agency felt that it needed to address the concerns about costs, we cannot say, but we did not feel that it was appropriate for the agency to allow the decision to be based solely on an advisory committee process that we thought reached its result on the basis of cost.

It is rare that the agency does not follow the recommendations of the advisory committee, which is the reason that the Chairman sent the letter, and we were pleased that the agency took the actions that it did. We want to be supportive publicly of that decision. We also think it is critical to work toward eventually closing the window. This is the goal that the FDA Commissioner himself stated at a November NIH conference. We must encourage companies to take incremental steps to get there. Clearly, the short-duration monoclonal antibody test was the first step that we needed to take in that direction.

We, as a society, talk about controlling medical costs, but we have not come to the point where we are making global decisions. With respect to the immediate decision about antigen testing, the criteria were that AIDS is a fatal disease, that we were able to stop some of its transmission, that there was a commitment on the part of the commissioner and the agency toward closing the window, and that we needed to take incremental steps.

There are definitely concerns with regard to the question of overall cost, because the statute does not address it and we have not yet reached the point in Congress, at least with the industries and the consumers approaching FDA, to say that one should consider changing the statute. It is a good question. I do not have a definitive answer, except to say that at the moment we have not addressed it as a society and, therefore, that the Congress has not addressed it.

Thomas Zuck: I would take issue with the observation that we have not addressed the health care cost question. Maybe the Congress has not, but those of us who are suppliers to hospitals and to the managed care organizations have been pressed to offer discounts and reduced prices. At the same time we are being asked to follow drug manufacturing practices, rationing and the like. So, mandating a test that costs 50 million or 60 million dollars for very little quality-life-years in gain is marginal at best. It is a very expensive endeavor, of nonspecific tests—replaced, that is, with new donors who are 13 to 16 times more dangerous than a repeat donor who has been screened multiple times. The cost is enormous, and the blood banks must absorb it.

William Sherwood: The American Red Cross's revenue as a supplier of blood products to the health care system is rapidly becoming capped. When new interventions come about and costs go up, they come as unfunded mandates. As a result, our revenues are squeezed, and so, to comply with the unfunded mandate, we must stop doing something else. In the selection of these mandates one must be very careful about whether it is going to be worthwhile in the larger view.

The Red Cross recently explained the new HIV antigen test to a group of hospital blood bank administrators. In the city of Philadelphia, with a usage of 350,000 units of blood per year, we will find one positive test result every 2.5 years. The hospitals' reaction was that they were not going to pay for that. As a result, we must fund the unfunded mandate. As a result, we will not do something else that we could have done.

Question from the Audience: Your remarks focused on the Blood Products Advisory Committee and its decision-making process. Can you describe how an advisory committee ought to work?

Anne Marie Finley: The Chairman recommended in his letter to Commissioner Kessler that BPAC be disbanded and that we start again with a national advisory committee on the safety of the blood supply. I personally believe, and here I am not speaking for Mr. Shays or for the committee, in greater representation; for example, a permanent voting member from CDC would be not a bad thing. We may want to raise the profile of BPAC beyond the level of just FDA. With regard to whether we want to make it a department level function, following through to some extent on the IOM recommendations, would be an option. We are interested in hearing the DHHS's response to those issues, recognizing that it has extensive technical expertise as well as a long history with BPAC.

The Chairman is a cosponsor of legislation that would require one-third of the voting membership of BPAC to be consumers or consumer representatives. That bill contains criteria that define *consumers*. Another bill, introduced by Porter Goss, defines *consumers* as individuals who have received blood or blood products or who represent blood or blood product consumer organizations. This is important; it was missing in the early 1980s. I do not think that anyone can say definitively that it would have made a difference, but Congress perceives that as something that many people feel comfortable with. That, again, goes to the consumer confidence issue. Perhaps it could be addressed by a greater voting membership on the part of the public.

DHHS Task Force on HIV and the Blood Supply

Mary Pendergast

When the Institute of Medicine (IOM) issued its report, *HIV and the Blood Supply* on July 13, 1995, the Secretary of the U.S. Department of Health and Human Services (DHHS) accepted it and stated that she agreed with the principles stated in the report and that details were to follow. She then asked Phil Lee, the Assistant Secretary for Health; David Satcher, the head of the Centers for Disease Control and Prevention (CDC); Harold Varmus, the Director of the National Institutes of Health (NIH); and David Kessler, the Commissioner of the Food and Drug Administration (FDA), as well as each of their deputies (Claire Broom at CDC, Ruth Kirchstein at NIH, and me at FDA), to convene to study the IOM report, to think about what it was saying, to take a hard look at what had happened between the time when the IOM report left off and today, and then to think about what, if anything, needed to be done in addition to or differently from what we had been doing in the past.

THE TASK FORCE CHARGE

Our charge is to respond to each of the recommendations made by IOM that might have moderated some of the effects of the AIDS epidemic. Because IOM had also urged the government and private organizations responsible for blood safety to evaluate their current policies and procedures to see if they fully addressed the issues raised by the recommendations, we are doing that as well.

As of the date of the Forum meeting, the task force had not completed its work. We have not yet prepared a report to the Secretary, although because the Secretary will soon testify before Congressman Shays on these very issues, I predict that we will finish the report sometime before she testifies.

We have spent quite a bit of time looking at the existing blood safety system. It comes as no surprise to any of you that things have changed in the 11 years since IOM saga left off. We are also looking at these very significant changes. We will be meeting with roughly 30 entities, including blood organizations, blood-related organizations, and persons or organizations interested in blood safety issues. These discussions will be part of our deliberations. At some point we will then make our recommendations to the Secretary, who will present them in testimony to Congressman Shays.

BLOOD PRODUCTS ADVISORY COMMITTEE

In the meantime, we have changed the composition of the Blood Products Advisory Committee (BPAC) somewhat, although it is important to recognize that we changed the composition of BPAC in response not to the IOM report but actually to a much earlier one. We had asked IOM to help us some years ago on our advisory committees, because one of the things David Kessler and I have been trying to do is make the agency more of a unitary organization. We have different product centers that sometimes operate with different plans, projects, and attitudes. They run their advisory committees very differently, so that we were not presenting a coherent picture to the outside world. It was causing some confusion.

Therefore, working with IOM, we addressed our advisory committee structure, and one of the things that we realized is that BPAC is constituted in a way that was very different from the way that the remainder of our advisory committees were structured. We began then to think about how we could bring BPAC into line with the rest of our advisory committees. It is seen as being reactive to IOM, but the goal actually was to make sure that there is more of a consumer voice on all of our advisory committees, to figure out ways to get the other federal agencies at the table, and to recognize that it is very hard to ask the people who are being regulated to make decisions that affect their economic interests. We had to come up with a new paradigm, and we have been striving to do that.

We are also trying to find other ways to develop a broad public conversation about the tough issues of the day. It is interesting to note how opinions about these things go in cycles. FDA used to have CDC and NIH on its advisory committee, until we were criticized as being too government focused and insular. Now we hear the call to put them back on again. We value their input. We agree that they must be at the table. We have been trying to figure out different ways to get CDC and NIH at the table. We do not want to be acting inconsistently, nor do we want to be acting alone. We need their advice and we need their consultation, but it is very challenging. Every agency has a full agenda; it is a great demand to ask them to take on not just their issues but ours as well.

DECISION-MAKING

Personally, I believe that it is critically important that we continue to talk about the issues, that we get all of the different points of view, recognizing that there is no such thing as a right or a wrong point of view, and that we at FDA know that many different vectors influence what we do. We must be very careful that we are not the "thought police," that we do not overvalue ideological purity, and that we have public forums and opportunities where people can say what they need to say in an open and forthright manner.

FDA has a tough job. The head of the FDA blood program must make specific decisions on a case-by-case basis when society does not have an agreed-upon paradigm for how to make those decisions. Therefore, the case-by-case decision-making drives the public policy, although ideally it should be the other way around. Blood is not alone in this. It is not uncommon for the case-by-case decision-making to outstrip the public policy, but we do not have a common set of values that is fully accepted by everyone. As a consequence, no one decision is perceived as being the right decision. As somebody said, "Which way are you going? Do you want more regulation or do you want less? Do you want the heavy hand of FDA to be greater or less? Do you want more safety or fewer costs?" I think that as a society we do not know what we want.

COST AS A FACTOR

With respect to whether cost is a factor, I do not think that it is, but it is also naive to think that absolute safety can be a reality. No product that FDA regulates, whether it is milk or human genome products, biotechnology, medical devices, or old-fashioned chemical drugs, is absolutely safe. If we strive toward absolute safety, we will drive the products off the market. We must accept that fact. The fact is, blood is not and is never going to be perfectly safe. It is as safe as we can get it, perhaps. It is as safe as blood anyplace in the world, but it is not absolutely safe. We are kidding ourselves, and we are kidding the public whenever we say that.

Therefore, given that fact, what do you do about it? Where do you draw the line? For every single product and every single therapeutic about which FDA makes a decision, we draw that line. In the summer if 1995 we had a situation in which a drug that prevents epileptic seizures in some people who are refractory to any other drug also gave 10 percent of them aplastic anemia. It is not safe, but it really makes a difference in some people's lives. Do we approve it or not? It is not safe, but it provides therapy, and we approved it. We approve things that are not safe every day of the week, and we always will; blood is not going to be any different. We must think of a new way to talk about blood, a way that is not kidding ourselves and kidding consumers. It is a risk-versus-benefit criterion, not a cost criterion. If you apply absolute safety, you are going to apply unlimited costs, and if you apply unlimited costs, then the heavy hand of FDA will make these products disappear. I do not know anyone who wants to see the United States without a blood supply, although that, in fact, is where we are headed if absolute safety is the paradigm that we are going to choose.

THE PUBLIC VIEW

Question from the Audience: The language of safety is somewhat misleading. Everyone knows that when we talk about automobile safety we are not completely safe. I am not sure we are as well informed about blood.

Mary Pendergast: For some FDA products the standard of safety is higher. For pesticides for foods that kids eat, the U.S. consumers want absolute safety. As for blood, U.S. consumers want absolute safety. We as regulators and you as industry and academics have helped to perpetuate that. It may be time to change the debate. There has never been an FDA official who has stood on Capitol Hill and said, "This drug is safe." Nobody ever says that. They always say that the benefits of this drug outweigh the risks. I know that the statute says "safe and effective," but you can only think of safety relatively. We are able to make the debate in some areas, but we have not made it in all areas.

Question from the Audience: You mentioned both the value of diverse opinions being expressed and an interest in continuing the dialogue. In what venues should that dialogue occur other than through the new BPAC and the coalition?

Mary Pendergast: It is fair to say that this has been our most fully debated issue. It is the nub of the question and is the toughest thing that we must deal with. I cannot yet tell you what we are going to do. Any suggestions are welcome.

V

Postscript

Investing in Regulatory Quality

Edward A. Dauer

What we have been exploring in our analysis of blood services regulation and its alternatives may be nothing less than good manufacturing practices for the law itself. What are the specifications of a good process for creating regulation and the procedures for ensuring compliance?

REQUISITES OF REGULATORY PROCEDURES

Predictability is certainly one of the requisites. There is also the challenge of matching the process to the problem in each of two dimensions. One is the dimension of effectiveness; the other is the dimension of efficiency. The procedure itself not only must work but it also must work better than any alternative in terms of its benefits and its costs.

On the one hand it has been argued that any good process must maintain science-based decision-making. On the other hand, it is stubbornly true that some of the necessary science will always be missing. It is not always possible to determine causation unambiguously, to "prove" that something is or is not in fact transmissible by blood. Under those circumstances, a good process may be one that is not frozen in place by the uncertainties and that does not allow uncertainty always to play the trump suit over other values such as public perception, morality, ethics, and economic welfare and the fact that every cost incurred in one endeavor inflicts additional risks somewhere else.

In addition, a good process would be one that minimizes disincentives and other adverse effects. It would not, for example, discourage innovation. It would not require that attention be paid to the method of compliance, as much as to the objectives of compliance.

PUBLIC PERCEPTIONS

A good process would be politically acceptable. It would have appropriate accountability and would achieve legislative goals in obvious ways.

In addition, leadership must listen and hear the articulated needs of the constituency. The constituency for many of these problems is the public. One of the needs of the public is their concern about the safety of the blood supply, and so a good process must in an irreducible way respond to that as well.

Could there be, however, a regulatory process that not only responds to the public's concerns about safety but that itself *promotes* the public's appreciation of the safety of the blood supply? People respond to risks in ways different from the ways in which medical science responds to risk; it is a challenge for us to take that into account. How can the public be brought to recognize the realities of safety so that in fact the decisions that are partly science-based, partly value-based, and partly economics-based can be the right decisions to be reached at the end of the day, not distorted by the politics of misperception and misinformation? This is the regulatory challenge.

What combination of private and public systems will accomplish these things? That is as difficult a question for those who dwell in the law side of the house as the medical issues about antigen testing and Creutzfeldt-Jakob disease are for those who live in the medical side. We do not have unambiguous answers either. Our knowledge about alternative procedures is itself indeterminate. For that reason, among others, the notion of a pilot project makes good sense.

It seems clear that some investment of time, energy, and thoughtfulness about these regulatory issues will pay a considerable dividend. After all, the regulatory process is the infrastructure within which all of these other problems come to rest. Government is art, and if the metaphor may be expanded, it is difficult to create a fine sculpture with a mean tool. Without an investment in the quality of the decision-making process itself, the odds of sculpting good decisions are not nearly as good as they might be.

Appendixes

A

Negotiated Rule-Making Procedure

[Added November 29, 1990]
5 U. S. Code §§ 561 et seq.

Preamble   The Congress makes the following findings:

(1) Government regulation has increased substantially since the enactment of the Administrative Procedure Act.

(2) Agencies currently use rulemaking procedures that may discourage the affected parties from meeting and communicating with each other, and may cause parties with different interests to assume conflicting and antagonistic positions and to engage in expensive and time-consuming litigation over agency rules.

(3) Adversarial rulemaking deprives the affected parties and the public of the benefits of face-to-face negotiations and cooperation in developing and reaching agreement on a rule. It also deprives them of the benefits of shared information, knowledge, expertise, and technical abilities possessed by the affected parties.

(4) Negotiated rulemaking, in which the parties who will be significantly affected by a rule participate in the development of the rule, can provide significant advantages over adversarial rulemaking.

(5) Negotiated rulemaking can increase the acceptability and improve the substance of rules, making it less likely that the affected parties will resist enforcement or challenge such rules in court. It may also shorten the amount of time needed to issue final rules.

(6) Agencies have the authority to establish negotiated rulemaking committees under the laws establishing such agencies and their activities and under the Federal Advisory Committee Act (5 U.S.C. App.). Several agencies have successfully used negotiated rulemaking. The process has not been widely used by other agencies, however, in part because such

agencies are unfamiliar with the process or uncertain as to the authority for such rulemaking.

§ 561. Purpose

The purpose of this subchapter is to establish a framework for the conduct of negotiated rulemaking, consistent with section 553 of this title, to encourage agencies to use the process when it enhances the informal rulemaking process. Nothing in this subchapter should be construed as an attempt to limit innovation and experimentation with the negotiated rulemaking process or with other innovative rulemaking procedures otherwise authorized by law.

§ 562. Definitions

For the purposes of this subchapter the term—

(1) "agency" has the same meaning as in section 551(1) of this title;

(2) "consensus" means unanimous concurrence among the interests represented on a negotiated rulemaking committee established under this subchapter unless such committee—
 (A) agrees to define such term to mean a general but not unanimous concurrence; or
 (B) agrees upon another specified definition;

(3) "convener" means a person who impartially assists an agency in determining whether establishment of a negotiated rulemaking committee is feasible and appropriate in a particular rulemaking;

(4) "facilitator" means a person who impartially aids in the discussions and negotiations among the members of a negotiated rulemaking committee to develop a proposed rule;

(5) "interest" means, with respect to an issue or matter, multiple parties which have a similar point of view or which are likely to be affected in a similar manner;

(6) "negotiated rulemaking" means rulemaking through the use of a negotiated rulemaking committee;

APPENDIX A

(7) "negotiated rulemaking committee" or "committee" means an advisory committee established by an agency in accordance with this Subchapter and the Federal Advisory Committee Act to consider and discuss issues for the purpose of reaching a consensus in the development of a proposed rule;

(8) "party" has the same meaning as in section 551(3) of this title;

(9) "person" has the same meaning as in section 551(2) of this title;

(10) "rule" has the same meaning as in section 551(4) of this title; and

(11) "rulemaking" means "rule making" as that term is defined in section 551(5) of this title.

§ 563. Determination of need for negotiated rulemaking committee

(a) Determination of need by the agency. An agency may establish a negotiated rulemaking committee to negotiate and develop a proposed rule, if the head of the agency determines that the use of the negotiated rulemaking procedure is in the public interest. In making such a determination, the head of the agency shall consider whether—

(1) there is a need for a rule;

(2) there are a limited number of identifiable interests that will be significantly affected by the rule;

(3) there is a reasonable likelihood that a committee can be convened with a balanced representation of persons who—

> (A) can adequately represent the interests identified under paragraph (2); and
> (B) are willing to negotiate in good faith to reach a consensus on the proposed rule;

(4) there is a reasonable likelihood that a committee will reach a consensus on the proposed rule within a fixed period of time;

(5) the negotiated rulemaking procedure will not unreasonably delay the notice of proposed rulemaking and the issuance of the final rule;

(6) the agency has adequate resources and is willing to commit such resources, including technical assistance, to the committee; and

(7) the agency, to the maximum extent possible consistent with the legal obligations of the agency, will use the consensus of the committee with respect to the proposed rule as the basis for the rule proposed by the agency for notice and comment.

(b) Use of conveners.

(1) Purposes of conveners. An agency may use the services of a convener to assist the agency in—

(A) identifying persons who will be significantly affected by a proposed rule, including residents of rural areas; and
(B) conducting discussions with such persons to identify the issues of concern to such persons, and to ascertain whether the establishment of a negotiated rulemaking committee is feasible and appropriate in the particular rulemaking.

(2) Duties of conveners. The convener shall report findings and may make recommendations to the agency. Upon request of the agency, the convener shall ascertain the names of persons who are willing and qualified to represent interests that will be significantly affected by the proposed rule, including residents of rural areas. The report and any recommendations of the convener shall be made available to the public upon request.

§ 564. Publication of notice; applications for membership on committees

(a) Publication of notice. If, after considering the report of a convener or conducting its own assessment, an agency decides to establish a negotiated rulemaking committee, the agency shall publish in the Federal Register and, as appropriate, in trade or other specialized publications, a notice which shall include—

(1) an announcement that the agency intends to establish a negotiated rulemaking committee to negotiate and develop a proposed rule;

(2) a description of the subject and scope of the rule to be developed, and the issues to be considered;

APPENDIX A

(3) a list of the interests which are likely to be significantly affected by the rule;

(4) a list of the persons proposed to represent such interests and the person or persons proposed to represent the agency;

(5) a proposed agenda and schedule for completing the work of the committee, including a target date for publication by the agency of a proposed rule for notice and comment;

(6) a description of administrative support for the committee to be provided by the agency, including technical assistance;

(7) a solicitation for comments on the proposal to establish the committee, and the proposed membership of the negotiated rulemaking committee; and

(8) an explanation of how a person may apply or nominate another person for membership on the committee, as provided under subsection (b).

(b) Applications for membership or committee. Persons who will be significantly affected by a proposed rule and who believe that their interests will not be adequately represented by any person specified in a notice under subsection (a)(4) may apply for, or nominate another person for, membership on the negotiated rulemaking committee to represent such interests with respect to the proposed rule. Each application or nomination shall include—

(1) the name of the applicant or nominee and a description of the interests such person shall represent;

(2) evidence that the applicant or nominee is authorized to represent parties related to the interests the person proposes to represent;

(3) a written commitment that the applicant or nominee shall actively participate in good faith in the development of the rule under consideration; and

(4) the reasons that the persons specified in the notice under subsection (a)(4) do not adequately represent the interests of the person submitting the application or nomination.

(c) Period for submission of comments and applications. The agency shall provide for a period of at least 30 calendar days for the submission of comments and applications under this section.

§ 565. Establishment of committee

(a) Establishment.

(1) Determination to establish committee. If after considering comments and applications submitted under section 564, the agency determines that a negotiated rulemaking committee can adequately represent the interests that will be significantly affected by a proposed rule and that it is feasible and appropriate in the particular rulemaking, the agency may establish a negotiated rulemaking committee. In establishing and administering such a committee, the agency shall comply with the Federal Advisory Committee Act with respect to such committee, except as otherwise provided in this subchapter.

(2) Determination not to establish committee. If after considering such comments and applications, the agency decides not to establish a negotiated rulemaking committee, the agency shall promptly publish notice of such decision and the reasons therefor in the Federal Register and, as appropriate, in trade or other specialized publications, a copy of which shall be sent to any person who applied for, or nominated another person for membership on the negotiating rulemaking committee to represent such interests with respect to the proposed rule.

(b) Membership. The agency shall limit membership on a negotiated rulemaking committee to 25 members, unless the agency head determines that a greater number of members is necessary for the functioning of the committee or to achieve balanced membership. Each committee shall include at least one person representing the agency.

(c) Administrative support. The agency shall provide appropriate administrative support to the negotiated rulemaking committee, including technical assistance.

§ 566. Conduct of committee activity

(a) Duties of committee. Each negotiated rulemaking committee established under this subchapter shall consider the matter proposed by the agency for consideration and shall attempt to reach a consensus concerning a proposed rule with respect to such matter and any other matter the committee determines is relevant to the proposed rule.

(b) Representatives of agency on committee. The person or persons representing the agency on a negotiated rulemaking committee shall participate in the deliberations and activities of the committee with the same rights and responsibilities as other members of the committee, and shall be authorized to fully represent the agency in the discussions and negotiations of the committee.

(c) Selecting facilitator. Notwithstanding section 10(e) of the Federal Advisory Committee Act an agency may nominate either a person from the Federal Government or a person from outside the Federal Government to serve as a facilitator for the negotiations of the committee, subject to the approval of the committee by consensus. If the committee does not approve the nominee of the agency for facilitator, the agency shall submit a substitute nomination. If a committee does not approve any nominee of the agency for facilitator, the committee shall select by consensus a person to serve as facilitator. A person designated to represent the agency in substantive issues may not serve as facilitator or otherwise chair the committee.

(d) Duties of facilitator. A facilitator approved or selected by a negotiated rulemaking committee shall—

(1) chair the meetings of the committee in an impartial manner;

(2) impartially assist the members of the committee in conducting discussions and negotiations; and

(3) manage the keeping of minutes and records as required under section 10(b) and (c) of the Federal Advisory Committee Act, except that any personal notes and materials of the facilitator or of the members of a committee shall not be subject to section 552 of this title.

(e) Committee procedures. A negotiated rulemaking committee established under this subchapter may adopt procedures for the operation of the committee. No provision of section 553 of this title shall apply to the procedures of a negotiated rulemaking committee.

(f) Report of committee. If a committee reaches a consensus on a proposed rule, at the conclusion of negotiations the committee shall transmit to the agency that established the committee a report containing the proposed rule. If the committee does not reach a consensus on a proposed rule, the committee may transmit to the agency a report specifying any areas in which the committee reached a consensus. The committee may include in a report any other information, recommendations, or materials that the committee considers appropriate. Any committee member may include as an addendum to the report additional information, recommendations, or materials.

(g) Records of committee. In addition to the report required by subsection (f), a committee shall submit to the agency the records required under section 10(b) and (c) of the Federal Advisory Committee Act.

§ 567. Termination of committee

A negotiated rulemaking committee shall terminate upon promulgation of the final rule under consideration, unless the committee's charter contains an earlier termination date or the agency, after consulting the committee, or the committee itself specifies an earlier termination date.

§ 568. Services, facilities, and payment of committee member expenses

(a) Services of conveners and facilitators.

(1) In general. An agency may employ or enter into contracts for the services of an individual or organization to serve as a convener or facilitator for a negotiated rulemaking committee under this subchapter, or may use the services of a Government employee to act as a convener or a facilitator for such a committee.

(2) Determination of conflicting interests. An agency shall determine whether a person under consideration to serve as convener or facilitator of a committee under paragraph (1) has any financial or other interest that would preclude such person from serving in an impartial and independent manner.

APPENDIX A

(b) Services and facilities of other entities. For purposes of this subchapter, an agency may use the services and facilities of other Federal agencies and public and private agencies and instrumentalities with the consent of such agencies and instrumentalities, and with or without reimbursement to such agencies and instrumentalities, and may accept voluntary and uncompensated services without regard to the provisions of section 1342 of title 31. The Federal Mediation and Conciliation Service may provide services and facilities, with or without reimbursement, to assist agencies under this subchapter, including furnishing conveners, facilitators, and training in negotiated rulemaking.

(c) Expenses of committee members. Members of a negotiated rulemaking committee shall be responsible for their own expenses of participation in such committee, except that an agency may, in accordance with section 7(d) of the Federal Advisory Committee Act pay for a member's reasonable travel and per diem expenses, expenses to obtain technical assistance, and a reasonable rate of compensation, if—

(1) such member certifies a lack of adequate financial resources to participate in the committee; and

(2) the agency determines that such member's participation in the committee is necessary to assure an adequate representation of the member's interest.

(d) Status of member as Federal employee. A member's receipt of funds under this section or section 569 shall not conclusively determine for purposes of sections 202 through 209 of title 18 whether that member is an employee of the United States Government.

§ 569. Role of the Administrative Conference of the United States and other entities

(a) Consultation by agencies. An agency may consult with the Administrative Conference of the United States or other public or private individuals or organizations for information and assistance in forming a negotiated rulemaking committee and conducting negotiations on a proposed rule.

(b) Roster of potential conveners and facilitators. The Administrative Conference of the United States, in consultation with the Federal Mediation and Conciliation Service, shall maintain a roster of individuals who have acted as or are interested in serving as conveners or facilitators in negotiated rulemaking proceedings. The roster shall include individuals from government agencies and private groups, and shall be made available upon request. Agencies may also use rosters maintained by other public or private individuals or organizations.

(c) Procedures to obtain conveners and facilitators.

> (1) Procedures. The Administrative Conference of the United States shall develop procedures which permit agencies to obtain the services of conveners and facilitators on an expedited basis.
>
> (2) Payment for services. Payment for the services of conveners or facilitators shall be made by the agency using the services, unless the Chairman of the Administrative Conference agrees to pay for such services under subsection (f).

(d) Compilation of data on negotiated rulemaking; report to Congress.

> (1) Compilation of data. The Administrative Conference of the United States shall compile and maintain data related to negotiated rulemaking and shall act as a clearinghouse to assist agencies and parties participating in negotiated rulemaking proceedings.
>
> (2) Submission of information by agencies. Each agency engaged in negotiated rulemaking shall provide to the Administrative Conference of the United States a copy of any reports submitted to the agency by negotiated rulemaking committees under section 566 and such additional information as necessary to enable the Administrative Conference of the United States to comply with this subsection.
>
> (3) Reports to Congress. The Administrative Conference of the United States shall review and analyze the reports and information received under this subsection and shall transmit a biennial report to the Committee on Governmental Affairs of the Senate and the appropriate committees of the House of Representatives that—
>
>> (A) provides recommendations for effective use by agencies of negotiated rulemaking; and
>> (B) describes the nature and amounts of expenditures made by the Administrative Conference of the United States to accomplish the purposes of this subchapter.

APPENDIX A

(e) Training in negotiated rulemaking. The Administrative Conference of the United States is authorized to provide training in negotiated rulemaking techniques and procedures for personnel of the Federal Government either on a reimbursable or nonreimbursable basis. Such training may be extended to private individuals on a reimbursable basis.

(f) Payment of expenses of agencies. The Chairman of the Administrative Conference of the United States is authorized to pay, upon request of an agency, all or part of the expenses of establishing a negotiated rulemaking committee and conducting a negotiated rulemaking. Such expenses may include, but are not limited to—

(1) the costs of conveners and facilitators;

(2) the expenses of committee members determined by the agency to be eligible for assistance under section 568(c); and

(3) training costs.

Determinations with respect to payments under this section shall be at the discretion of such Chairman in furthering the use by Federal agencies of negotiated rulemaking.

(g) Use of funds of the Conference. The Administrative Conference of the United States may apply funds received under section 595(c)(12) of this title to carry out the purposes of this subchapter.

§ 570. Judicial review

Any agency action relating to establishing, assisting, or terminating a negotiated rulemaking committee under this subchapter shall not be subject to judicial review. Nothing in this section shall bar judicial review of a rule if such judicial review is otherwise provided by law. A rule which is the product of negotiated rulemaking and is subject to judicial review shall not be accorded any greater deference by a court than a rule which is the product of other rulemaking procedures.

B

Workshop Participants

WORKSHOP ON RISK AND REGULATION
January 23–24, 1995

Lew Barker
Efficacy Trials Branch
Vaccine and Prevention Research
  Program
Division of AIDS NIAID, NIH

Celso Bianco
Vice President Medical Affairs
New York Blood Center

Penny Chan, Ph.D.
Commission of Inquiry
Blood Systems in Canada
Toronto, Ontario

Harry W. Chen
HemaSure Corporation
Marlborough, MA

Eileen Church
Communications Manager
American Association of Blood Banks

Marcia Crosse
Program Evaluation and Methodology
  Division
U.S. General Accounting Office

Jacqueline D'Alessio, Ph.D.
U.S. General Accounting Office

Leonard I. Friedman
American Red Cross
Holland Lab

Elizabeth Goss
Fox, Bennett & Turner
Washington, DC

Harold Kaplan, M.D.
University of Texas
Southwestern Medical Center

Kurt R. Kroemer
U.S. General Accounting Office

Jan Lane
American Red Cross

Karen Shoos Lipton
CEO
American Association of Blood Banks

Jane Mackey, MBA
Topeka Blood Bank, Inc.

James MacPherson
Executive Director
Council of Community Blood Centers

John McCray
HemaSure Inc.
Marlborough, MA

Brian McDonough
American Red Cross
Arlington, VA

Charles Mosher
Blood Centers of America, Inc.
E. Greenwich, RI

Jean Otter
Director of Regulatory Affairs
American Association of Blood Banks

Mary K. Pendergast
Deputy Commissioner and
 Senior Advisor to the Commissioner
Food and Drug Administration

Barbara Peoples
American Red Cross
Holland Lab

Mark Philip
IMMUNO US, INC.
Rochester, MI

Beatrice Pierce
National Hemophilia Foundation
Rancho Santa Fe, CA

William H. Portman
The Institute for Transfusion Medicine
Pittsburgh, PA

James Reilly
Executive Director Director
American Blood Resources Association

Miriam Sparrow, Esq.
New York Blood Center, Inc.

Edwin Steane, Ph.D.
ICCBBA

Eugene Timm
IMMUNO US, INC.
Rochester, MI

Peter Tomasulo, M.D.
TM Consulting, Inc.
McLean, VA

Lee Ann Weitekamp
The Blood Center of Southeastern
 Wisconsin
Milwaukee, WI

WORKSHOP ON
MANAGING THREATS TO THE BLOOD SUPPLY
September 21–22, 1995

Lew Barker
Efficacy Trials Branch
Vaccine and Prevention Research
 Program
Division of AIDS NIAID/NIH

Patricia Bezjak
Chief Operating Officer
Metropolitan Washington Blood Banks

Celso Bianco, M.D.
Vice President/Medical Affairs
New York Blood Center

APPENDIX B

Irene Church
American Association of Blood Banks

Brian P. Conway, Esq.
Bayer Corporation

Richard J. Davey, M.D.
Chief Medical Officer
American Red Cross

Rob Dickstein
Director, Regulatory Affairs
Pall Corporation

Sandra Ellisor
Ortho Diagnostic Systems, Inc.

Susan Frantz-Bohn
FDA/CBER
Division of Congressional and Public Affairs

Steve Friedman
Dechert, Price, & Rhoads

Eric Goosby
Office of HIV/AIDS Policy

Elizabeth Goss
Attorney
Fox, Bennett & Turner

William J. Hammes
Associate Counsel
Bayer Corporation

Harriet Newman (MT) ASCP
Donor Advocate
Virginia Blood Services

Nancy Newman
Knapp, Petersen & Clark

Jean Otter
American Association of Blood Banks

Stephen Redhead
Analyst Congressional Research Service
Library of Congress

James Reilly
Executive Director
American Blood resources Association

Paul Schmidt, M.D.
Head, Transfusion Medicine
Transfusion Medicine Academic Center
Florida Blood Services

Toby Simon, M.D.
President and CEO
Blood Systems, Inc.

Harold C. Sox, Jr., M.D.
Chairman, Dept. of Medicine
Dartmouth-Hitchcock Medical Center

Miriam Sparrow, Esq.
New York Blood Center, Inc.

Jane Starkey
Deputy Director
Council of Community Blood Centers

Ron Welborn
Community Bioresources, Inc.

Edward Wolf
Sr. Associate General Council
American Red Cross

Sam Wortham
Group Vice President
Pall Corporation

C

Acronyms

ACUS	Administrative Conference of the United States
AIDS	Acquired Immune Deficiency Syndrome
ARC	American Red Cross
AABB	American Association of Blood Banks
ABRA	American Blood Resources Association
CAP	College of American Pathologists
CBER	Center for Biologics Evaluation and Research, Food and Drug Administration
CCBC	Council of Community Blood Centers
CDC	Centers for Disease Control and Prevention
CFR	*Code of Federal Regulations*
CLIA	Clinical Laboratories Improvement Act
CJD	Creutzfeldt-Jakob Disease
EPA	Environmental Protection Agency
FAA	Federal Aviation Administration
FACA	Federal Advisory Committee Act
FDA	Food and Drug Administration
FD&C	Food, Drug, and Cosmetic Act
GMP	good manufacturing practices
HIV	human immunodeficiency virus
NIH	National Institutes of Health
OSHA	Occupational Safety and Health Administration
PDUFA	Pharmaceutical Drug Users Fee Act
PLA	Product Licensing Application